Don't Just Be Alive...LIVE!

Naturally Restoring Your Maximum Human Potential

I0442066

Don't Just Be Alive...LIVE!

Naturally Restoring Your Maximum Human Potential

By
Dr. David Adams, DPSc, DC, FICPA

ISBN: 978-1523976096

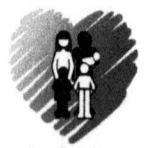

Family Focus Wellness Center
www.familyfocuswellnesscenter.com

Dedication

I dedicate this book to Ashley Kate, a beautiful little girl who never learned to walk or talk, yet taught me more about joy and living life than anyone I ever met. I miss you, Ash. XMO Forever 8

Acknowledgements

First and foremost I would like to thank my Creator for giving me life and blessing me with a career that allows me to make an impact in this world.

To my family, Trish, Blake, Allie, and Ashley for being the ever-present part of my life that makes it worth living.

To my mother and father for giving me the support and opportunities to pursue my passion, which have allowed me to improve the lives of so many, young and old.

To all the teachers, instructors, professors, and doctors who have educated and mentored me over the years, molding me to be the doctor, teacher, mentor, and coach I am today.

To all the thousands of patients I have had over the years who have taught me so much more than I ever learned in school.

To my staff who has helped support our mission of helping people improve their quality of life and relationships.

A special thank-you goes to Dr. Chess Miles, Dr. Melvin Aldridge, Dr. Chester Graham, and Dr. Brad Aylor for always being there to support and encourage me every step of the way.

Contents

CHAPTER FIVE

Introduction

Can you get healthy just by reading a book about health?

Of course not. There's no way a book can make you healthy, no more than I could read a book about flying an airplane and call myself a pilot.

Would you get in a plane with me at the controls?

I should certainly hope not.

As you read through the following pages, I want you to spend some time getting into your mind, to get in-between your ears. The vast majority of people who pick up health books and read them are trying to find out *how* to be healthy, but the simple truth is that it's more important to discover *why* you must do it.

Every diet known to mankind — the ones that you've heard of, the ones that you've tried, the ones that didn't work for you — did work for somebody, and they didn't work for somebody else.

Why is it that while one person is diagnosed with cancer and told they're going to die in six weeks, it happens exactly as predicted while the person next to them with the same diagnosis is still alive thirty-five years later?

In the following pages, we are going to spend a lot of time exploring how to get healthy. More importantly, we'll answer why you need to. If you understand the why behind the how, then you can have true success and long-term results.

This book helps you understand the importance of:

- Breaking commonly held belief systems
- Knowing why the things you've been doing haven't been working
- Learning what you can do that works
- Knowing your own role in your healthcare
- Seeing how your belief systems and actions are much more important than the suggestions given to you by your specialist
- Recognizing or realizing that the power to heal is within you
- Opening your eyes and recognizing that the system has failed you
- Seeing that if you want different results, you have to do something different

We have to understand how to confidently step out of a broken healthcare system and begin to make an impact in our own lives and our own families.

I've started reading hundreds of books over the years, but I rarely finish them, because I usually find that everything I need to know is contained in the first five chapters. This book is intentionally only five chapters long because I want you to get the meat and potatoes, and skip all the fluff and stuff. My intent is for it to be action-packed, full of quality information, and only 150 pages.

I encourage you to get through all of the pages; however I suggest that you don't read it all at once. It can be read in a very short period of time, but as stated earlier, reading a book doesn't make you healthy, and it can't make you a pilot.

So I would like you to break this book down into bite-sized pieces, and really spend time contemplating, absorbing, and applying the concepts to your life. When I guide practice members using this approach, we take six months to go through this short book. We do that because we know that to have extremely successful outcomes, we need to break it down to small, bite-sized pieces.

There's an old saying:

How do you eat an elephant?

One bite at a time.

I know you can eat, or read, this book in one bite, but I also know that it will not have much of an impact if you do it that way. In order to get the best results out of this process, read no more than one section per week. After you read the section—which should take you only a few minutes—spend the next week thinking, contemplating, praying, and otherwise soaking in the content of that section. Then take the individual action steps that are in that particular section. You'll get much more out of the process if you do it this way.

My hope for each and every reader is that reading this book doesn't just become an academic exercise, but that reading it instead becomes truly life-empowering. My hope is that you share this with your family members and your friends. Perhaps you enlist an accountability partner or a group that goes through the process together. It has been shown again and again that results are much better when we are involved with other people. I recall having a workout partner who would meet me at 5:30 in the morning. On those mornings that I didn't want to wake up and go out there, I would get up and do it anyway, because I didn't want to leave him waiting for me.

My hope is that you understand, apply, and share the concepts, so that you not only empower yourself and get more out of life, but you also help your family members and your friends to do the same.

CHAPTER ONE

What Is Your Why?

If you're going to be alive, you might as well live.

Here is the story of how I found my Why. In the fall of 2008, I found myself sitting in one of those little vinyl recliner chairs that you see in all hospital rooms. I was sitting by my daughter, who recently had four organs transplanted, then developed lung cancer as a side effect of the medications she was on.

Ashley was on a ventilator at the time, and I remember watching her chest rise...pause...fall...pause...then rise again, as the ventilator machine pumped life-sustaining oxygen into her tiny body. We were sitting in a hospital 704 miles away from home, where my wife and my daughter had been living for nearly two years.

I remember looking at my wife and saying, "We didn't put her through all this so she could be alive, but so that she could live."

I flew home.

We started to talk about, "How are we going to get her out of the hospital and get her home?"

I remember, sometime within the next week, my thirteen-year-old son said, "Hey, Dad, let's go outside and hit some balls."

We had a batting cage in the backyard for him; he's an excellent baseball player.

I looked at him and said, "I don't feel like it," and I crawled in bed and watched TV the rest of the night.

The next morning, I woke up, looked in the mirror, and realized I was a lousy father. I also recognized that I wasn't being the best husband I could be, and I wasn't the best friend, uncle, son, brother, employer, or any of the other relationships I had in my life. In that moment, I recognized that if I truly want to take care of my children, I have to take care of myself. If I truly value the people I say I care about, then I have to first take care of me.

All of the stress of my family being broken and my daughter being sick and in the hospital room so many miles away had caused me to not take care of myself. Then it hit me.

I remembered what I had said about my daughter, "We didn't put her through all this so she could be alive, but so she could *live*."

I realized that I wasn't living, either. In that moment living more for me, for my wife, and for my kids became my Why. I decided in that moment that just being alive was not enough. It was time to start *living*. I share this story because it was in that moment of looking in the mirror that I began to see the world differently.

I began choosing to live more. I changed my lifestyle to help my family and to help myself live more. I changed the way I work and I began mentoring my practice members rather than just treating their signs and symptoms. I started putting together programs to teach them to live more.

I became that doctor who does spend more time with their patients to help them really understand how to put more living back into their life. I saw my practice members feel better and live life more fully. That is what I want for you as well. I want you to find your Why so you too can start living life more.

> *I am so excited to get started. I have been looking for someone who does Functional Wellness. This is my new chance for a fresh start. My best friend has been in your program for four months and if I get half the results she has, I know it will change my life.*
>
> *~ Amanda J.*

THIS BOOK IS FOR YOU

I don't want this to be just another health book that you read and then put on your shelf, saying to yourself: *Oh, that was full of really nice information.*

I have written this book to help people take action and make a change. The bottom line is that if we want different results, we have to do something different. My hope is that this book is a little bit different than anything you've read before. I want you to take it out of your head and into your life, and really act on the information that you'll be reading. This book is not designed to be purely cerebral or academic; it's designed to challenge you to step outside of the rut that you're currently in.

Reading and using the information in this book will help you:

- Create a new lifestyle
- Create new habits
- Create new thought processes that will transform you

- Move to the next level

Sick and Tired

Every day in my professional practice, I meet people who come in with all manner of conditions, symptoms, named diseases, and problems.

The true problem is when those conditions begin to have a negative impact on your life:

- The conditions interfere with your ability to enjoy life.
- They interfere with your ability to make the most of your relationships.
- You get tired.
- You get worn out.
- You have less energy.
- You don't really have the opportunity to fulfill the purpose that you're really here for.

Sure, you get up and experience life, but so many people are just going through the motions of the day. They tell me they get up, they do what they have to do, they go to bed, and can't fall asleep. Maybe they do fall asleep and wake up through the night, only to wake up not rested the next day to do it all again. They're not really experiencing the joys of life, the wonder of life, the enrichment that life has to offer us.

Does this describe you?

Are you tired of being tired?

Are you worn out and run down and ready for something different?

Are you ready for that transformational experience?

When you take radical steps, you get radical results. I'm going to challenge you, as you read through the coming pages, to think about action steps that you're going to take that can make a radical change in your life.

You can be that person that other people look to and say:

"Wow, I can't believe that you lost eighty-three pounds!"

"Wow, I can't believe that you reversed your conditions or diseases without taking the medications!"

"I can't believe that you used to be diabetic and now you're not!"

"I can't believe that you were brave enough to go out and try something different, and create a new you!"

Are You Ready?

One of the hardest parts of restoring your life, your health, your vitality, and reconnecting with your thoughts, your actions, and your mindset is getting started. Often people ask me for help quitting smoking.

"Absolutely, I can do that, yes," is my answer.

The first question I ask them is, "Do you want to quit smoking?"

If the answer is no, then I tell them that we're done, because there's absolutely nothing that I can do to help them quit smoking until they decide that it's time.

The same thing is true for regaining our health and our vitality. Somebody else can't do this for you. You have to be ready.

How do you know if you're ready?

- You're worn out and tired.
- You're just sick of the experiences that you're having now.
- You want a difference in your life.

If you feel this way, consider it already done.

In your mind's eye, see the result on the back end that we've already actually accomplished.

You have it within you! You have the strength. You have the ability. Don't you dare tell yourself that you don't have the willpower. Your body is self-healing, and it will do its part.

You just have to make the decision that you are ready to take action. Don't worry about having all the answers. You're not going to have all the answers right away. It's going to take some time. It's a journey and a process. You need to allow yourself to take that first step, because taking that first step is the hardest part.

My team and I have coached thousands of people through the process. If you ask, we are going to be here to support you. The following chapters are going to educate you. As you learn more and become more informed, you'll find it easier and you'll become more enthusiastic about the process and eventually have stronger and stronger desires to make more and more profound changes.

No One But You Can Do This

When most people arrive at the doctor's office, it's with the expectation that their healthcare provider is going to fix them. Most people see their healthcare as a series of events.

There was that time when I was younger when I fell off the swing set and broke my arm. I went to the doctor and they put my arm in a cast. Maybe you've had an ear infection and took some antibiotics and the ear infection went away. Or maybe you've had a heart attack and had surgery to get stents put in. In situations like these, people see their health as a series of events, rather than as a process.

Health is a process, and you are the one who is in control of that process. There is no better doctor in the world than Doctor You. You have the healing capacity within you, and you are the one in charge of your healing.

One of the biggest challenges in healthcare is that patients are lacking education. Unfortunately, in today's healthcare climate, the average doctor's visit lasts only seven to nine minutes.

You may have become accustomed to sitting down with your doctor, looking at your labs, and hearing the doctor say, "This is high. This is low. Here's your meds, I've got to go." The next thing you see is their back as they are heading out the door to give their next patient seven to nine minutes.

You are left sitting there wondering what just happened and what you are supposed to do.

You get your medications, you go home and start taking your pills, and six months later, you go back for a lab test only to find that things have gotten worse because you weren't taught about what you can do.

Only about 3 to 5 percent of your health is due to your genetics, which means about 95 to 97 percent depends on lifestyle choices. If you know how to live a healthy lifestyle, and you apply it to your life, then your choices can affect 95 to 97 percent of your health. That means you can expect a big change — a huge difference — when you improve your lifestyle.

Mentoring is often missing from healthcare. This book shows you how to put that back into your healthcare routine.

> *I have seen nine doctors in the last three years for my female problems and none of them could find the cause of my excessive bleeding. Since being on your program and taking your advice I no longer have an issue. My periods are back to normal and the best part about it is I am off of all the drugs that were making me feel so lousy. Thanks for showing me how to change my lifestyle to change my life. Oh yeah, I have already lost sixteen pounds.*
> *~ Missy M.*

WHY DEFINE YOUR WHY?

Why are you still reading this book?

Why are you interested in this topic?

What is it you want to accomplish?

What's important to you?

In order to have a truly successful experience in regaining your health, you really have to understand why you're doing it.

When I was twenty-eight years old, I got a phone call at 3:17 in the morning.

My mother was frantic on the other end of the line, saying, "Your father just had a heart attack. We're headed to the hospital."

I immediately jumped out of bed and rushed to the hospital, only to find my dad lying there looking extremely vulnerable. I've always respected my dad. He's always been very strong, and yet at that time he looked very weak. He looked very sad. He looked very out of control. This wasn't the father who raised me.

I recall talking to him.

He said, "Son, you remember that your grandfather died at fifty-three from a heart attack. I'm fifty-three, and I just had my first heart attack. Get ready, because in another twenty-five years, this is where you're going to be."

I never spoke back to my dad; that's not the relationship we had. I always had respect for him.

But I remember looking at him, and even as a young man of twenty-eight, with all the conviction in me—I don't know where it came from—I looked at him and I said, "No it's not, because I have twenty-five years to make better choices than you made."

At the age of twenty-eight I had found my Why. I wasn't going to put my children through that same situation as a fifty-three-year-old man. I was going to be there for them, as well as for my grandkids and my great-grandkids. I never knew my grandfather. My entire relationship with him exists within a single photo of me as a one-year-old sitting on his lap. I've never gotten to know the man, but I've heard stories of how much I would have loved him. My Why is that I'm going to be there for my as-yet unborn grandkids, and eventually great-grandkids.

What is *your* Why?

For You

I meet people all the time who are ready to make a change. They're ready to feel better, but often, they feel guilty about taking time for themselves, investing time and finances into their own health. I especially see this to be true with mothers. Mothers are so good at taking care of everybody else that they often put themselves last.

You have to understand that taking care of you doesn't make you selfish. Putting yourself first doesn't mean that you're putting others last.

By taking better care of yourself, you're now better equipped:

- To take care of your spouse
- To take care of your family
- To be a better family member
- To be a better friend
- To be a better employee or employer

If you take care of yourself, you can have a bigger impact on those you care about and those you love. So please don't fall into the trap of believing that you need to put yourself last and everybody else before you. By not taking care of yourself first, you end up having less of yourself to share with those you love. It's not selfish to put yourself first. In fact, it's selfless, because taking care of yourself makes you a better caregiver to those you love.

For Your Family

One important reason for you to take exceptional care of yourself is so that you can take better care of your family. I married my beautiful wife twenty-two years ago, and I intend to be with her until death do us part. I don't want to spend the last ten, fifteen, twenty years of our lives with her changing my diapers or emptying my bedpan. It's important to me that we get to spend those vital decades enjoying life, enjoying the fruits of our labors, enjoying our retirement, enjoying each other, hopefully having grandkids or great-grandkids, and being there spending quality years with our family.

All too often in our society, as we get older the expectation is that we will be prescribed seven, ten, twelve, even *seventeen* different medications. It is typical to be spending time not with our families, but instead spending that time going from this doctor to that specialist, and jumping around from one doctor to the other.

Often the conversations of elderly people revolve entirely around:

- What health condition they have

- What doctor they're seeing
- What they're asked to do or have to do according to the doctor
- What specialist they're referred to

I would much rather hear the elderly talk about what vacation they just went on or what their grandkids are doing. These are certainly the conversations I want to be having as I get older.

Ultimately my goal is to end up in a motor home, not a nursing home. The motor home represents freedom. Maybe a motor home isn't for you, but I think we can all say that as we enter our golden years that we'd like them to be golden, full of freedom, full of energy, full of vitality—not full of doctors visits, hospital stays, nursing homes, and bedpans.

Studies show that over 75 percent of Americans are going to end up in a nursing home. Of the remaining 25 percent, many will never have the energy or vitality to enjoy the freedom of the motor home. When you're in your elderly years, you don't get to make that decision. You get to make that decision with the choices you start making today. I challenge you to be one of those few who get to fully enjoy their elder years. Choose today that you will be one of those few, for yourself and your family.

> *I really just can't believe how great we feel! We are spending more time with each other and with the kids.*
> ~ *Jason and Tammy D.*

Your Contribution

We have a very sick society. We have a very sick culture. We have a culture of worn-out, worn-down people. If you turn on the news, you're going to see a lot of bad news. You're going to see a lot of negative stuff. You're going to see a lot of problems, a lot of despair, a lot of broken things. Our society is worn down, sick, and broken because so many of us as individuals are worn down, sick, and broken.

If you as an individual are worn out, sick, and broken, you're not able to contribute as well—not only to yourself and to your family; you certainly can't consider making an impact on others. If you are interested in making an impact, it has to start with you. You have to get your own house in order. Then you can take the concepts that you're learning and help apply them to your spouse and your family.

Once you have that in order, you can contribute to your community, state, nation, and the world. If you truly want to make an impact—and I believe that we all should—then you have to understand that you can't do it unless it starts at home, with you. This is why

I don't want you to feel guilty about taking care of yourself. By taking care of yourself, you're going to be able to make a bigger impact on your community and the world.

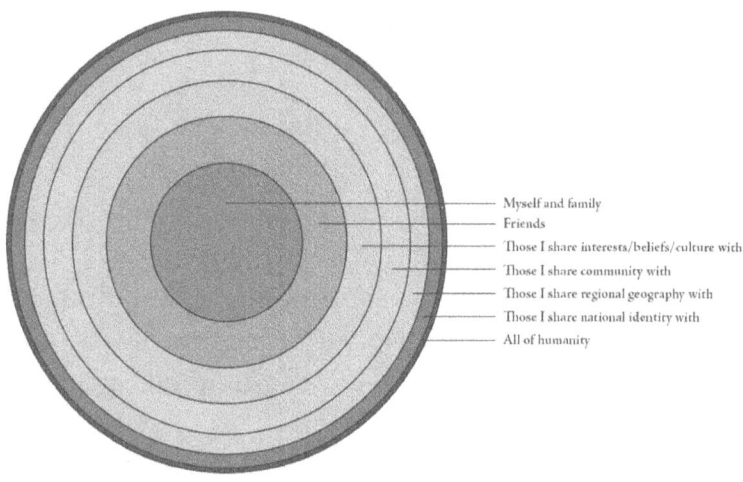

Myself and family
Friends
Those I share interests/beliefs/culture with
Those I share community with
Those I share regional geography with
Those I share national identity with
All of humanity

Why define your Why?

So many people ask, "How do I do this? How do I do that?"

People overlook the more important questions, "*Why* am I doing this? *Why* am I doing that?"

If you have an event coming up, and you want to look great in that outfit, you can go on a diet and lose ten pounds, but most likely—we've all done it, we all know—you're probably going to gain twelve or thirteen back. However, if you decide that you want to be there for your kids, be there for your spouse, and be there for your future generations, you have started to define your Why.

If you want to lose ten pounds so you look cute in a dress, you can achieve those temporary results. But if you want to be there for your grandkids and your great-grandkids, you have to truly define that Why, so that you can make lasting changes.

Lasting changes come from defining your Why, not from, "How do I do this program, diet, exercise, etc.?"

So often I hear people say, "I don't have the willpower," or, "I did really good for a few months and then fell off."

If you want lasting results, taking time to define your Why is one of the most important things you can do.

I WANT TO BRAINWASH YOU

I want to brainwash you. That sounds absolutely ridiculous.

It sounds crazy, doesn't it?

But the vast majority of Americans have already been brainwashed into believing that we have a healthcare system that can make us healthy. What we call *healthcare* is a disease management system, and it is failing us miserably!

I want to take some time to de-brainwash you, to help

you understand that you are your best physician. You care about you more than any doctor you've ever been to. You are completely capable of creating that optimal lifestyle that you desire.

> *I feel younger and healthier than I have in years. My body is looking like I want it to and my digestive symptoms have completely disappeared. Thank you for putting all the pieces together in a simple and easy-to-follow system that I can apply. I have to say that my wife's hormones appear to be balancing out as she is a lot easier to be around. Don't tell her I said that. I have seen her try every diet out there and this is the first time she is truly seeing results. Thanks for helping her; she is my world.*
>
> *~ Randy R.*

Have You Turned On Your TV Lately?

Do you have trouble sleeping?

Do you struggle with insomnia?

Do you feel like you are not getting a full night's rest?

Now you can finally do something about it with DECEIVA. With Deceiva, you can finally get that good night's sleep you have been looking for. Deceiva can easily correct the problem and finally give you that great night's rest that you deserve. Deceiva is not for everyone. Side effects may include nausea, dry mouth, itching, difficulty breathing, and diarrhea. Additional side effects may include nightmares, drowsiness, hallucinations, and electric shock sensations. Other more severe side effects include cardiac arrest, liver failure, or even death. If you should happen to die stop taking Deceiva and contact your doctor immediately.

Ask your doctor if Deceiva is right for you.

Deceiva: Because we can get away with it.

How many times have you seen an ad like this?

Many, many ads promise feeling wonderful and feeling great, but end in, "Ask your doctor if (drug name) is right for you." Then we hear the fast talker at the end of the commercial reading that long list of side effects and problems that the drug may cause.

A recent study done in Seattle showed that for every $1.00 spent on prescription medications, there's $1.85 spent on treating the side effects of those medications. We've seen the exact same thing in our own office. The vast majority of our practice members eliminate about 80 percent of their symptoms just by decreasing or eliminating the medications that they're on. These drug commercials have brainwashed us into believing that there's a pill for every ill; the solution for every symptom is another drug. The reason that there are drug commercials is because they work! People do go to their doctors and they do ask for drugs like Deceiva. Commercials sell a lot of drugs. We've been brainwashed into believing that the solution to our health problems is taking more medications.

We Do What We Do Because That's What We've Seen Done

We're relational beings, and we tend to behave much in the same way as the people around us. Therefore, our behaviors and our choices become very similar to the people who surround us. Wealthy people hang out with wealthy people. People who like sports hang out with people who like sports. Health nuts hang out with other health nuts.

Have you ever met somebody new and then caught yourself sounding like them or having the same mannerisms as them, maybe using some of the same language or phrases?

This has to do with how we're neurologically wired. If it's always been modeled to us that drugs are the solution, then that's what we're going to turn to. If it's been modeled to us that exercise is a good thing, then we're probably pretty good at exercising. If it's been modeled to us to take time off and have vacations, then we probably do that. If our parents worked and never took a vacation, then that's probably what we do.

"Why Do We Cut Off the Ends of the Roast?"

Another way that we were brainwashed was within our own homes. We pretty much do what our parents did. I'm reminded about the old story about the roast, in which a young lady is learning to cook. Her mother is showing her how to cook a roast, and she cuts the two ends off the roast before she places it in the pan, covers it up, and puts it in the oven.

She asks her mom, "Why do you cut the ends off the roast?"

Mom says, "I'm not really sure. That's just the way that your grandmother always did it. Why don't you call her?"

So she calls the grandmother and asks, "Why do you cut the ends off the roast?"

Grandma replies, "I'm not sure. That's the way my mom always did it. Why don't you call her?"

So the young woman calls her ninety-eight-year-old great-grandmother and asks her, "Granny, why do you cut the ends off the roast?"

Granny responds, "Honey, the roast wouldn't fit in my pan!"

In the 1990s, scientists spent a lot of time trying to map the human genome. It was commonly believed that we are just a collection of our genes. It was thought that if your grandma had diabetes and your mom has diabetes, well, then, you are going to have diabetes.

What the research shows us is that the cause of diabetes is about 95 percent due to your lifestyle, and only 5 percent is genetics. So if you had modeled for you a lifestyle that produces sickness, illness, and disease, then you should expect sickness, illness, and disease.

However, you can break that cycle! It's imperative that you do, not just for you, but for your children, your grandchildren, and your great-grandchildren. If you can break that cycle and model healthy decisions, healthy behaviors, and healthy action steps, then you are going to end up in that motor home. Just because it's always been done a certain way doesn't mean it's always been done right. You don't have to do it that way.

Chapter One Action Items

1. Navigate to
   www.familyfocuswellnesscenter.com/testimonials
   Watch some testimonials and get inspired by the progress
   so many others have achieved. Understand that the only
   difference between you and them is that they took the
   first step and got started.

2. Navigate to
   www.familyfocuswellnesscenter.com/live Print and then
   fill in the "Chapter One: What is Your Why?" worksheet.

3. Share your answers with someone else. Remember
   we are much more accountable and therefore much
   more successful when we involve someone else and
   ask for their support. If you need help filling out the
   worksheet, or if you want us to review your answers,
   or if you have any questions, email me at dradams@
   familyfocuswellnesscenter.com.

CHAPTER TWO

The Way We Experience Healthcare Is All Wrong

You are the first doctor I have been to who has taken the time to help me find out what is really going on. I have been on so many drugs that covered up my symptoms. It is refreshing to know that I don't need them. I feel better than I have in years!
~ Jessica P.

THE SYSTEM IS BROKEN

It's time to take the pulse of our healthcare system so we can understand how it's working, or not working.

When you don't feel well or get sick, you go to the doctor or healthcare provider, and they typically do things like take your temperature, take your pulse, take your blood pressure, maybe test some reflexes, in order to diagnose what underlying condition you have. To really understand how you've gotten to where you are, in this chapter we're going to be trying to really diagnose the healthcare model that most of us are currently experiencing.

It's time to check the health of healthcare. We have to start with the word *healthcare*. We don't have a healthcare system in this country. In actuality, we have a disease management system. Recently I heard a doctor from the renowned Cleveland Clinic saying that most physicians have never even had a healthy patient before.

How can we call it healthcare, if we don't actually enter into the system until after we're sick, until after we have symptoms?

We should call it what it is, which is a disease management system. We have a system based on a model called *fee for service*. Fee for service rewards doctors and physicians for doing services. The only way to be paid is to have sick patients that need services. This isn't healthcare; this is disease management.

There are two hospitals in my town; both have tripled in size in the last fifteen years. If we were truly advancing in healthcare, then that would never happen. True healthcare should be causing the system to become smaller, and instead we've seen it bloating considerably in the last several decades.

Let's Check the Health of Our Healthcare System

If we want to check the health of healthcare, we have to see the results that we're getting for the dollars that we are spending. As of July 2014 (the most recent data available), the United States is spending $2.8 trillion on healthcare. And expenses have continued to rise every year since. That is $2.8 trillion dollars annually, or an average of $8,915.00 for every man, woman, and child in this country. The average dollars spent on healthcare in the rest of the developed world is around $3,000.00 per person. We have to ask ourselves what that additional 66 percent we are spending is actually getting us.

The United States has the most expensive and least effective healthcare system in the world. We spend $300 billion on pharmaceutical drugs. That's almost as much as the rest of the world's medicine spending combined.

"The healthcare system is unsustainable. We're spending almost twice as much in America as any other country on Earth. We're really mortgaging the future. Not just the health of healthcare — we're talking about the health of the nation."

— Dr. Don Berwick
Head of Medicare/Medicaid, 2010–2011

"Our forefathers in medicine were really about patients. It was about a passion for healing, and when medicine became a business then we lost our moral compass. I think we've gotten into a great deal of trouble because of that."

— Dr. Steven Nissen
Chairman, Cardiovascular Medicine
Cleveland Clinic

"When you reward physicians for doing procedures instead of talking to patients, that's what they're going to do—procedures."

—Dr. Leslie Cho
Cardiologist, Cleveland Clinic

"Roughly 75 percent of healthcare spending goes to treating preventable diseases."

—Centers for Disease Control

"Thirty percent of healthcare costs (roughly $750 billion annually) are wasted and do not improve health."

—Institute of Medicine

"Approximately 187,000 people die each year from medical errors and hospital-acquired infections. That is over 512 people per day lost to medical errors. Based on these numbers, it is the third leading cause of death. When you consider instances where medical errors cause some form of *harm* but not necessarily death, the incidence rate may be as high as 40,000 per day."

—Health Affairs
Centers for Disease Control and Prevention

"If trends continue through 2020, up to ⅕ of healthcare spending, or up to $1 trillion annually, will go to treating the consequences of obesity."

—RAND Corporation

"On balance... the benefits that [the] U.S. healthcare currently deliver[s] may not outweigh the aggregate health harm it imparts...."
— *Journal of the American Medical Association*

Did you catch that last quote?

According to the *Journal of the AMA,* healthcare in America may be causing more harm than good. That's astonishing! One of the best ways to prevent dying unnecessarily is to stay away from hospitals. This is one of the reasons why I'm so passionate about sharing the information in this book with you. This book may save your life!

As you can see, the healthcare system is really sick: It's broken. It's failing us. We can no longer afford to put our faith in this system.

> *I have learned so much that is empowering me to make better choices. I don't know why they didn't teach me this when I was diagnosed with type 2 diabetes. They just prescribed me Metformin. Now, my blood sugars are under control and I have already been able to get off of three of my meds.*
> *~ Dustin M.*

How Did We Get Here?

As you can see, healthcare is a mess.

How did we get here in the first place?

At the turn of the twenty-first century, there were many health disciplines that were all somewhat on the same playing field. Medical doctors, chiropractors, osteopaths, homeopaths, naturopaths, acupuncturists, and a few others all played on relatively the same field.

- They were all equal in stature.
- They were equal in dollars spent.
- They were equal in how people used them.

However, at around the same time, some started to really market pharmaceuticals. Drugs began to take over the marketplace, and we started to believe that we could have better health through lab-based research. The research produced some pretty amazing medications that really made some significant difference in people's lives. However, they also made a tremendous amount of money, which meant pharmaceutical companies had to find new symptoms and new problems, so they could use these newfound medicines. Essentially, the corporate medical lobby came to the different factions trying to convince practitioners to prescribe more and more medicines.

The medical doctor went that route, and if you think about it today, there are basically two things that medical doctors do:

1) They prescribe medications.
2) They do surgeries.

Outside of that, there are not a lot of tricks in the bag. Gone are the days of the family doctor who would come to your house, show you the things that you've been doing wrong, coach you, or explain to you how to regain your health. Now it's all about masking your symptoms so that you feel better, regardless of how much your disease is destroying your health.

The chiropractors said, "No, we're a drug-free healing art, and we're going to continue to be that way."

The American Medical Association went after them and tried to shut them down—actually going all the way to the Supreme Court in the Wilk case. In the decision, the Supreme Court reprimanded the AMA for the actions they had taken against the chiropractors, all because the chiropractors didn't want to prescribe drugs.

The osteopaths said, "Yeah, we'll take the medications and begin prescribing drugs, but we still want to be osteopaths."

There still are some osteopaths, but they're few and far between, and mostly indistinguishable from medical doctors, meaning they are primarily dispensing more and more drugs.

Those who decided to stick to their roots and not prescribe medicine—homeopaths, naturopaths, acupuncturists, and others—have been marginalized in today's quick-fix, feel-good-while-actually-getting-sicker, disease management system.

Where Will This Lead Us?

So where are we going?

If we continue down this road it will lead to even more and more prescriptions with more and more side effects. If we understand that the system is broken, and we recognize that doing more of the same thing is going to get us more of the same results, then it's time that we do something different.

Ask yourself:

Are there more people with cancer, or diabetics, or people with heart disease than when I was a kid?

Are there more children suffering from allergies, asthma, autism, ADD, ADHD?

Are there more children with obesity?

Disease rates have skyrocketed and at the same time the cost of so-called healthcare has skyrocketed as well: if we keep doing the same things, we're going to continue to get the same results. Chronic sickness and illness for all. As you've seen, it's not looking too good for our disease management system.

If we want to break the status quo we have to learn to take individual responsibility for our actions. We're going to have to learn to step out of that broken disease management system. That's what this book is all about. The takeaway is: we're going to have to step out of that system—for you, your family, and your loved ones. If we want true health, we have to demand healthcare, not settle for disease management.

WHAT'S IN A NAME?

We have been conditioned to believe that it's really important to know what we have. If we have a sick plant, and the leaves are turning brown, most of us would immediately think perhaps it needs water, or perhaps it needs some sunlight or fertilizer.

However, when it comes to our own health, if we have a wilting or a sick human, our initial thought is: *I wonder what I have.*

So we rush off to WebMD, and we put all our symptoms in the symptom checker, because what we're looking for is a diagnosis.

Our second thought is usually: *I wonder what I need to take.*

Why do we automatically think this way?

We've all seen those commercials on TV where they have the people that are not so happy, and they describe all their symptoms, and then the next thing you know, the parents are chasing the children out in the front yard. All they had to do was take the medication being advertised.

We hear all the virtues of the medication, only to hear the fast talker at the end say, "May cause headaches, nausea, itching, allergies, an unsafe drop in blood pressure, rapid breathing, rapid heart rate, infections, rash, diabetes, diarrhea, constipation, digestive problems, liver damage, and death."

But all the commercials end with, "Ask your doctor if this medication is right for you."

Drug companies have spent billions and billions of dollars to convince us that this is the way that we should think; we've been conditioned to believe that what's important is the name of the disease, the diagnosis. The treatment is always either another drug or another surgery. In order to have a wonderful healthy life, what we need to understand is that the diagnosis we receive doesn't really matter. What really matters is what we decide to do about it.

I don't want you to get stuck on, "What do I have?"

That's the least important thing you need to know about your health.

What's more important is to ask yourself: *What am I going to do to improve my condition?*

Your diagnosis is not something to get hung up on.

Rather, it's better to focus your time, effort, and energy on, "What can I do differently to get a different outcome?"

Where you are relative to your health is nothing more than the result of the choices and the decisions that you've been making. If you want to be somewhere else, if you really want to get to the underlying cause of your conditions, then you have to recognize that it's time to *do something different.*

> *This is the first time in years that I have not suffered with the approach of a storm system. No stiffness, no joint pain, no headaches, just beautiful rain! Thank you again. I look forward to continued improvement and spreading the great results! Have a great weekend.*
>
> *~ Lyn J.*

Your Diagnosis Doesn't Matter

Many people, especially as they get older, tend to talk about what diagnosis they have:

"I have heart disease."

"I have cancer."

"I have diabetes."

"I have a thyroid problem."

The name of the disorder is the least important aspect of correcting it. Most health problems come from the same underlying cause, which is the inability of your body to adapt to whatever stress it is dealing with.

So the resolution to almost all health problems is to help your body adapt to the true underlying stress that is causing your condition.

The diagnosis is so much less important than, "What am I going to do about it?"

This book helps you focus your energy on the healing process, and on the choices you can make, and how those choices affect your diagnosis. The purpose of this book is to discuss how we can correct the underlying cause of health problems, not merely cover up or mask your symptoms. If you want to be healthy then you must focus less on what the name of your problem is and more on how you are going to deal with it.

Are you suffering from CDD—Conditioned Disorder Disorder?

Most Americans are. We have been so conditioned to believe that when we get sick, fall ill, or otherwise don't feel well, we need to go see our doctor to find out what's wrong with us. We've been conditioned to believe that the answer can be found in getting a diagnosis and taking medications.

If you want to transform your body, your health, and your life, then you *must* understand this:

The answers to your problem cannot be found outside yourself.

There is no magic lotion, potion, or pill. You will never find it. If you're ready to take your life back, you have to start by curing your CDD, so let's get started.

A recent study showed that up to 20 percent of us are misdiagnosed annually. That is over 64,263,000 of us who are misdiagnosed each and every year. There is a one-in-five chance you don't have what your doctor says you have. One of the problems with just looking at the name of the disease is that all the testing that you will get will be related to that diagnosis and all the drugs you are placed on are tied to that diagnosis.

What if the diagnosis were wrong?

Medical Necessity

What makes something medically necessary?

Unfortunately, it's usually not your doctor who makes that decision; rather, it's your insurance carrier, a third-party payer, making that decision. Those decisions are based upon the name, or the diagnosis. If the name or the diagnosis is the most important thing, then the testing is all going to be around that particular diagnosis. As the insurance companies have become more involved in our healthcare decision-making, many fewer things are considered medically necessary.

For the insurance companies, it's all about maximizing profitability by spending less and less on their customers. Another way to look at it is that your doctor is getting a lot less information with which to determine the direction of your care.

Medical necessity is typically a judgment that's made by someone sitting behind a computer, often with only a high school education and zero clinical experience, in an office a few thousand miles away. It's been taken out of your doctor's hands.

If you want to restore your health, you have to do proper testing. Often those proper tests aren't deemed medically necessary.

If it can help you, and if it can help your doctor determine the true underlying cause of the problems, would you consider that medically necessary for you?

I sure would and I certainly think you should too.

Cigna HealthCare's definition of medical necessity for physicians is:

> …healthcare services that a physician, exercising prudent clinical judgment, would provide to a patient for the purpose of evaluating, diagnosing, or treating an illness, injury, or disease, or its symptoms that are: a) in accordance with the general accepted standards of medical practice, b) clinically appropriate in terms of type, frequency, extent, sight, and duration, and considered effective for the patient's illness, injury, or disease, and c) not primarily for the convenience

of the patient or physician, or other physician, and not more costly than alternative services or sequence of services at least as likely to produce equivalent therapeutic or diagnostic results as to the diagnosis or treatment of that patient's illness, injury or disease.

(This can be interpreted to mean, if there is not a cheap drug to treat it, then it's not medically necessary.)

In reading that definition, did you read anything about healing?

Did you read anything about creating optimum function or wellness?

The entire definition was built around the concept of treating an illness, injury, or disease, or symptoms, but said absolutely nothing about what's in the best interest of helping you create your optimum function, if you felt lousy before the diagnosis and the disease made you feel even worse. The doctor can only help you get back to feeling as lousy as you did before you were diagnosed. Optimum health and function are never part of the insurance companies' plans. If you are relying on your insurance to help you get healthier, then you are going to be in a world of hurt.

> *We are so excited you did the testing that you did. My wife has been suffering for years and you are the first doctor to take the time to tell us what is really going on with her and lay out a plan to fix it. Thanks.*
>
> ~ *Cecil L.*

The Underlying Cause Is What's Important

Imagine that one of your children is not doing very well in school. You know she's a bright child but her grades seem to be slipping lately. Suddenly, you find your child coming home with Cs, and then Ds, and eventually, she's getting Fs.

You could say, "Well, Allie, I know that you sit next to Abby in school, and Abby's very bright. She's very smart, and she makes good grades, so I want you to cheat off of Abby the rest of the year."

Sure enough, Allie is obedient, so she cheats off of Abby for the rest of the year. Allie's report card comes out. She's getting straight As. That's great!

So are you going to give her a little gold star and praise her and tell her how great she is for making straight As?

Are you going to become parent of the year for telling your child to cheat?

Or, in actuality, did you make things harder on her?

What's going to happen next year, when Allie's not sitting next to Abby, and she's not prepared?

Now she's in Algebra 2, but she didn't learn anything in Algebra 1 because she cheated her way through. You have set her up for failure.

Does this sound like a familiar approach when it comes to your healthcare?

For many it should, because this is what you're doing when you take medications to mask your symptoms. Perhaps you feel better, or you have numbers that look better on your blood labs, but in actuality, all you've done is set yourself up to allow that underlying condition or stress to continue to get worse while you and your doctor celebrate better numbers on your labs.

What you really have to do is focus on the problems, not just cover up the symptoms.

Maybe it takes a little more time, but instead of teaching your child to cheat for the good grades, you could sit down with your child, and ask, "Allie, what's going on at school? Why are you struggling?"

Maybe if you spend enough time and ask enough questions, you'll discover that she's being bullied. Perhaps the kid behind her has been stabbing her with a pencil or stealing her lunch money so she hasn't eaten lunch in the last six weeks. You really need to get to the underlying cause of the problem. In this case, the underlying cause was the bully.

What's the underlying cause of your health problems?

If you want to be well that's what you and your health team need to find out.

If the "Check Engine" light comes on in your car, what would you do?

Most of us would ignore it for a day or two, but if it didn't go away, we would probably take it to a mechanic. If that mechanic hooked your car up to the computer, cleared the trouble code, and gave you your car back and the "Check Engine" light was off, you'd probably feel pretty good about it. You would pay your bill and drive on home.

If while you were driving home, the "Check Engine" light came back on, what would you do?

You'd probably get a bit frustrated, turn around, and go back to that mechanic and ask him to check it out. He'd put it on his computer, clear the trouble code again, and get that light out and send you home. The next day, the "Check Engine" light comes back on.

How many times would you go back to the same mechanic, who obviously isn't getting to the underlying cause of the problem?

What if that mechanic pulled out a piece of duct tape

and put it over the dashboard so you could no longer see the light?

Would that fix the problem?

I don't think so. What you'd really have to do is find a mechanic who would be willing to dig a little deeper and find the true underlying cause of the problem, so that your engine doesn't give up while you're driving down the road.

If you want optimal health you need to find a doctor who's willing to work with you to find the true underlying cause. Not one who prescribes more and more meds to mask your symptoms.

DON'T BE AFRAID TO BE INDEPENDENT

At what point did we allow or invite our doctors to make all of our healthcare decisions?

At what point did we forget that we are in control of our own bodies?

Far too many people have been brainwashed to believe they can't make a decision concerning their health or their body without first consulting their medical practitioner.

I recall helping a practice member of mine who was on twelve different blood pressure medicines. After having a conversation with her, she wanted to decrease the amount of medication she was taking, but was afraid to because this is what her doctor had prescribed. We set her up on a program to restore her health and improve her nutrition, and she quickly found that she was being overmedicated, and her blood pressure was bottoming out.

One time she actually was taken to the emergency room in an ambulance because the medications caused her blood pressure to drop dangerously low. It wasn't long after that incident that we had a conversation in which, with tears in her eyes, she told me she was going to have to drop out of our program. Her doctor actually told her that if she were going to continue working with me and improving her health, the doctor would no longer continue to be her doctor.

I had to help this practice member do some self-reflection and recognize that if she was taking twelve blood pressure medicines, something was wrong with her treatment. If her blood pressure was bottoming out, then obviously it meant she was on too much medication. It was very difficult for her to make the decision to leave her doctor of so many years, but ultimately she had to do what was in the best interest of her health. I worked with her and we found her a different medical doctor who could provide for her needs, someone who wanted to improve her situation. Within one year she was off all twelve blood pressure drugs, as well as three different cholesterol-lowering drugs. We were able to help her get her life back.

I want you to recognize that you are your best doctor. You are the one who can make the best choices for yourself and your family. Our doctors should be consulted for their opinions and their knowledge; however, that should be filtered through what we learn on our own. Nobody's going to take as good care of you as you are.

> *You taught me it's okay to want more than the status quo.*
> *Thank you!*
>
> ~ *Mekela P.*

Your Doctor Doesn't Always Know Best

There are many knowledgeable and well-trained physicians and specialists who know how to care for their patients. Although they've spent a lot of time and effort and want to help their patients, the time they spend with their patients is getting slimmer and slimmer. Most people are finding that they spend less time with their healthcare providers. If you're like the average person who goes to see their provider for seven to nine minutes every six months or year, it's a little bit ridiculous to think that they know more about you than you do. After all, you have spent every day with yourself since birth!

You know yourself better than anybody else in the world. You're there for every little sniffle and sneeze;

you're there for every little ache and pain. Sometimes it's difficult in that seven- to nine-minute window with your physician to relay what's really going on.

You should listen to your doctor's opinion, and listen to their advice, and if it makes sense and if it falls in with what you were thinking, then by all means follow it. However, if you don't feel one hundred percent comfortable with their advice or their recommendations, I absolutely would not follow their advice. I would suggest that you get a second opinion, or a third opinion, or a fourth opinion. I would suggest that you spend some time researching and studying.

There's so much information available to you that you should be checking these things out prior to making life-impacting decisions. I know it frustrates a lot of doctors when their patients come in and they've got a lot of information on a topic, but we've all heard the horror stories of people getting the wrong kidney removed or having surgery on the wrong hip. In the United States alone, more than 2,000 people a year are getting surgeries on the wrong body part. I don't want you to become one of those horrific statistics. Use your doctor's expertise and experience as a tool in your tool chest; however, don't assume they always know best.

Drugs Aren't Always the Answer

Most people are familiar with getting an infection and taking a round of antibiotics. Usually the infection goes away. Medicine has proven itself to be very beneficial in certain circumstances. However, in a quest to expand limitless market share and sell more and more drugs, our culture has come up with a medication for every potential symptom.

There's simply not a medication for every problem. For example, if you break an arm, you might take some pain medication temporarily. If it hurts enough, it's a very good idea to take the medication for a short period of time, but that pain medication certainly isn't going to heal the arm. However, if the bones are set, aligned properly, and held in a cast, the body will perform a miracle. Over the next three to four months, it will lay down new bone tissue and heal that bone.

Health and healing come from within us, they do not come from external sources. Although occasionally there is a time or a place for a medication, what we have to understand is that that time or that place should be reserved for emergency, short-term care.

If you have high cholesterol, your doctor can put you on cholesterol-lowering medication, which can certainly lower your cholesterol, but it does absolutely nothing to address why your cholesterol became high in the first place.

To experience optimal health, we need be proactive and look for:

"What's the underlying cause of my signs or symptoms?"

Instead, many people stop at:

"Can this medication give me a quick fix?"

You Are Your Own Best Doctor

Did you know?

- Out of the approximate 100 trillion cells that make up your body, about 90 percent of them are bacteria, viruses, and other microorganisms. Only about 10 trillion cells actually belong to you.

- A red blood cell will circle your entire body about 4,320 times each day.

- With every breath, your ribs are set in motion to the tune of over 120 million individual rib motions per year.

- The average human heart will beat 2.8 billion times in its life. Image a car that could drive 2.8 billion miles.

- There are fewer people in the world than bacteria in your mouth right now.

- If you counted one brain cell per second, it would take you more than 3,171 years to count them all.

- Your brain is more powerful than your Smartphone and computer combined.

Your body is an amazing creation that's capable of completing the most complicated tasks with ease. If your body is capable of doing such amazing things, it's certainly capable of taking care of so many of the problems that we present to our doctors' offices, if given a chance or given the proper support.

As you can see, your body is capable of so many astonishing things.

Don't you think it is capable of healing most ailments?

Your body has the capacity to:

- Lower your blood pressure
- Reverse your diabetes
- Eliminate your body pain
- Balance your hormones
- Fix your thyroid
- Eliminate your joint pain

I remember when my children were younger and they would get sick. I always loved it—now hear me out on this—I enjoyed that when they got sick they were more cuddly and they wanted to snuggle. We never took our kids to the pediatrician and got them antibiotics. They never had any. But we had many conversations in which I would explain to them that inside their bodies they had little armies of cells whose only job was to fight the bad guys that were making them sick.

How cool is it that your body can do that while you're sleeping?

It can find all the little bad guys, and it can destroy them, so that in the next two or three days, you're going to be feeling a lot better.

Rather than telling my kids, "Oh, you're sick? I'm so sorry. Take this medication," they got a story that really helped them learn and appreciate the fact that their bodies were self-healing and self-regulating.

All too often in our culture, we say to a child, "Oh, your ear hurts? Take these pills. It will make you feel better." Then we say, "You have a headache? Here, take these pills. It will make you feel better." Then we say, "You've got a sore throat? Here, take these pills. It will make you feel better."

Then when our children are adolescents and they get dumped by their first puppy love, and a friend comes along and says, "Oh, here, take this. It will make you feel better," or, "Oh, smoke this, and it will make you feel better," we are shocked and surprised that our children would. We are angered that they would do something so stupid.

Could it be that we conditioned them to believe that drugs make them feel better?

Could it be that this nations drug problem is a result of our cavalier over use of prescription drugs?

Decades ago, alcohol and marijuana were the gateway drugs. Unfortunately for many kids today, the gateway drugs are coming from the family medicine cabinet.

Chapter Two Action Items

1. Reflect on your past experience with healthcare. Was it health *care* or disease management?

2. Navigate to www.familyfocuswellnesscenter.com/live Print and read "Health Care vs. Disease Care" and fill in the attached worksheet.

3. Share your answers with someone else. Remember we are much more accountable and therefore much more successful when we involve someone else and ask for their support. If you need help filling out the worksheet, or if you want us to review your answers, or if you have any questions, email me at dradams@familyfocuswellnesscenter.com.

CHAPTER THREE

Ninety-Nine Percent of Your Health Happens Outside Your Doctor's Office

> *Thank you for holding me accountable to your process. I know I couldn't have done it on my own. I tried; it didn't work. This works. Thank you and thank your team for me. You guys are great!"*
>
> *~ Ben C.*

YOUR CHOICES MATTER

Look at where you are now.

Consider all the areas of your life, including:

- Health
- Spiritual connection
- Relationships
- Hobbies
- Activities
- Career

Are you happy?

Your choices have determined where you are. If you're happy with where you are, then you need to continue to make choices similar to the ones that you've been making. If you're not completely satisfied with where you are, then you need to understand that changing your mind, making different choices, and taking action *will* change your results.

This chapter is about learning to trust yourself, trust your intuition, and learning to understand that the decisions that you make determine where you are now and where you'll be in the future.

Listen to Your Intuition

We live in a culture where science is king. We believe if it hasn't been proven, then it's not a fact. We don't believe anything unless it's a scientific fact, but our common sense and intuition tells us there are so many things we could never design a science experiment to prove.

In science, the gold standard is the peer-reviewed, double-blind study. Many believe if the research hasn't met that criteria, then it won't work. In 2003, The *British Medical Journal* published an article entitled, "Parachute use to prevent death and major trauma related to gravitational challenge: systematic review of randomised control trials." It was a scientific review of the literature on the efficacy of a parachute.

The research showed that there had never once been a peer-reviewed, double-blind study of whether a parachute will prevent major trauma related to gravitational challenge. We've never taken a group of people and pushed them out of an airplane with parachutes and compared them to another group of people pushed out of an airplane without parachutes to see if using a parachute is a good idea. But we universally accept that if we're going to jump out of an airplane, we'd better have a parachute! In its conclusion, the study states, "As with many interventions intended to prevent ill health, the effectiveness of parachutes has not been subjected to rigorous evaluation by using randomised controlled trials."[1]

Our intuition tells us that having a parachute is obviously a pretty good idea. We don't have to have some researcher in a white coat in a science lab somewhere, telling us that we should not wear a parachute because its effect has never been proven through study. Our own eyes just tell us that it works. Common sense is one thing that has been dismissed in healthcare. I think it's time that we bring it back.

[1] http://dx.doi.org/10.1136/bmj.327.7429.1459
(Published 18 December 2003)

> *I have dealt with thyroid problems for over thirteen years and was sick and tired of never seeing the changes I wanted. I heard from a friend of mine about Dr. Adams and how he used a different approach. I attended his talk, "Why Your Lab Tests Could Be Normal but You Still Have Thyroid Symptoms," and I am so glad I did. I have been able to turn my health around and get the relief I had been seeking for thirteen years. And I was able to get off my meds as I found the true underlying cause of my symptoms. If you have a thyroid problem I highly recommend you attend Dr. Adams' talk. You won't regret it.*
>
> ~ *Jen R.*

Your Choices Define Your Results

The circumstances we find ourselves in are nothing more than the result of previous choices we've made. I don't know how to play a piano because I never took piano lessons. However, if I wanted to be a piano player, I could choose to find piano teachers in my town. I could choose to call them. I could choose to make an appointment to take lessons. If I made these choices consistently and often enough, the outcome would be that in a year or two, I might be able to be a pretty good piano player.

Do you think I could take a seven- to nine-minute lesson once or twice a year and be a good piano player?

Probably not.

Then why do we think that if we spend seven to nine

minutes once or twice a year talking to our doctor that we will ever be truly healthy?

If you want different results, you have to do something different. So many people continue to gripe and moan and complain about the circumstances they are in while continuing to make the same choices that put them in their circumstances.

The only way to get different results is to do something different, and the only way to do something different is to make a different choice and then take action.

Most people think the only healthcare choice is to go see a medical practitioner, who typically offers one of two solutions:

1) They give you medications and drugs.
2) They suggest surgery.

There are lots of different specialists with techniques and high-tech tools and gadgets. But it all comes down to one of two things:

1) More medications
2) More surgeries

If you want a different result, you have to do something different. You have to look outside of that current medical model and find people who are doing something different. If you look in the right place you will find people who are getting different outcomes and different results.

Is there a friend whom you consider to be very healthy, maybe healthier than you?

They spend less money on healthcare than you. They get better outcomes than you do. They have healthier families and friends than you. Maybe it's time to stop and ask them what they are doing differently.

See if you can recognize differences between how you and your friend:

- Exercise
- Eat
- Shop
- Get healthcare
- Choose friends
- Relate to family

Taking Time for You Is Not Being Selfish

When consulting with my new practice members, it's often the case that they are so busy taking care of other people, they don't take care of themselves.

They'll use an excuse like:

"I can't invest that money in me because I have to have that money for my spouse."

"I have to have that time for my child."

"I'm already taking care of my adult parents."

Many feel a sense of guilt about taking time for

themselves, but you have to recognize that if you don't take care of yourself, then you can't really take very good care of your spouse, your children, your aging parents, or whoever else might rely on you.

How you feel determines how you act. If you feel run down and worn out, then you're probably not going to be much fun to be around. If you feel full of youth, vitality, and energy, then you can invest more of yourself into your relationships.

Remember at the beginning of Chapter One, I shared that I felt like a lousy father because I didn't want to go outside and hit some balls with my son?

I realized that if I value the people I say I care about then I have to first take care of me.

> *My wife is a patient of yours. I just wanted to say thank you for giving her back to me. Since beginning your program, she is feeling so much better and we are getting along so much better. She looks fifteen years younger and is acting that way too (wink wink), if you know what I mean. Keep up the good work. You are changing lives.*
>
> ~ *Justin B.*

YOUR DOCTOR IS ONLY ONE OF THE TOOLS IN YOUR TOOL CHEST

Imagine a carpenter shows up at your house and brings only a hammer. He can't be very effective if that's the only tool that he has in his tool chest. For many people, when they get ill, the only tool in their tool chest is their medical doctor or the clinic that they frequent. Now imagine equipping that carpenter with a full complement of wrenches, sockets, screwdrivers, sanders, saws, hardware, lumber, and so on. He'd have everything he needs to build a proper house.

This section explores how your doctor's recommendation should be just one of many tools in your healthcare tool chest.

Building Your House

Let's say that there are two people standing on the road, looking out on an empty plot of land. They each decide to build a house. They're going to be neighbors.

The neighbor on the left finds a good, reputable homebuilder in the area to build. The neighbor on the right calls around until the cheapest contractor can be found.

Then the reputable contractor finds a reputable concrete company to lay the foundation. The neighbor on the right finds the cheapest concrete contractor.

The contractor for the left neighbor hires good carpenters to erect the walls and build a solid roof, and the neighbor on the right finds the cheapest ones. They use the cheapest lumber, drywall, and shingles.

From the road the houses are going to look very similar.

When it's moving day, the neighbors move in and everybody's happy. However, the house on the left is going to weather the storms better. It's going to hold up to the roughhousing of the people inside better. The first time it hails, its roof holds up, whereas the one on the right starts to leak. The house on the left lasts decades while the one on the right shows signs of wear and tear in just a few short years.

In the long run with upkeep and maintenance and all the wear and tear that will occur, the neighbor in the house on the right is going to have to put up a ton more money to replace the drywall, get the electric fixed, redo the plumbing, and buy a new roof.

Picture how you treat your body compared to the construction of these houses. You are a collection of the raw materials that you place in it, which is mostly going to be food and drink. If you're eating good, high-quality foods and nutrients, in the short run, it may cost a little bit more — just as the house on the left cost a little bit more.

When your body is nothing more or less than a sum of all the materials or the raw ingredients that you bring to the mix, it's important as you focus on restoring your health that you bring in *quality* raw materials.

Are you building a shack that constantly requires work, or are you building a strong temple?

Building a Solid Foundation

When I speak to groups, one of the questions I often ask is, "What do I have to do if I want to be healthy?"

The most common answers are to:

1) Eat right
2) Exercise

These two things are certainly very important; however, these two things are kind of like a roof. A roof on my home is very welcome and very important, but you have to have a solid foundation and frame to place that roof upon or it's not going to work very well.

Can you imagine a homebuilder showing up at an empty lot with only shingles as the first building materials?

I would be looking for a new contractor, one who has the concrete trucks showing up first to build a solid foundation.

I meet people all the time who say, "Well, I've done this nutrition program, and I've done that system, and I've counted calories, and I did all kinds of things, and all I did was gain weight."

I meet other people who say, "I worked out really hard, and I did this kind of exercise, and then I joined this gym, then I got a personal trainer, and I never really got any solid results."

The reason for their lack of results is that nutrition and exercise are kind of like the roof of the house. They didn't get results because they were trying to build the roof before they laid a solid foundation.

If you want to be healthy, you have to lay that foundation. In your health, the foundation is good, proper brain function.

Symptoms that indicate your brain is not functioning well can include:

- Low energy
- Fatigue
- Brain fog
- Forgetfulness
- Anxieties
- Depression
- Mood swings
- Hot flashes
- Insomnia

The brain is your foundation because the brain controls everything else.

Well-functioning and balanced hormones are also important players in your health. If your hormones are out of balance, then you're going to have some significant health challenges.

Poor hormone balance causes:

- Cravings
- Stubborn weight gain
- Lack of libido.

Your mom said, "You are what you eat."

She was almost correct. You are what you keep and what you absorb. I often meet people who say that they're eating good, healthful diets, but they're still gaining weight or still having health challenges. Even if you are eating the right things, if you don't have good, proper gut health, you don't have a good-functioning liver, gall bladder, pancreas, and digestive system, you are likely to still have many health problems. A poorly functioning digestive system can cause you to gain weight, even while eating all the right things.

If you are spending tons of money doing different nutrition or eating programs, but your digestive health isn't ready for it, you're really just throwing your money away and wasting your time. You're probably also getting pretty frustrated.

Poor digestive health can cause:

- Acid reflux
- Heartburn
- Bloating and gas
- Burping
- Bad breath
- Poor brain health

To lay a proper foundation, you have to make sure that you have:

- Good brain function
- Proper hormone balance
- A good, solid purification program to restore your liver and digestive system

> *These last twenty-one days have changed my life! I have so much energy and feel better than I have in years. The first three days were rough, but I am so glad you challenged me to do this for myself and my family. I would never have done this on my own. Thank you, Dr. Adams. Oh yeah – I lost nine pounds and another four since I finished the program.*
>
> *~ Kelly W.*

Building a Leak-Proof Roof

Now that you've laid a solid foundation, you can build your roof. In terms of your health, the roof consists of proper nutrition and exercise. When it comes to nutrition, many of the things that you've been taught are bad for you are actually good for you, and many of the things that you were taught are good for you are actually quite bad for you.

Essentially, nutrition is not that difficult. We need to eat more of the things that God makes, and eat fewer things that humans make. It's really as simple as that. We shouldn't be eating things from boxes or bags or cans, we should be eating things that are fresh.

A good rule of thumb is that if you can set it out on the countertop, and it doesn't rot, it's probably not good for you. If you laid a steak out on your counter and forgot to cook it and went to bed, by morning you would know that that thing was not edible.

On the other hand, I remember finding a Jolly Rancher while cleaning my dad's garage. It had been there for fifteen years. I was able to take it out of the package and just eat it, and it tasted the same. If a food doesn't rot after fifteen years, chances are that eating it is not very good for you.

Many people and many diet programs get hung up on counting calories, or counting carbs, proteins, or fats. However, most of us want to live in the real world and eat real food. The key word is *real*. I've found very few people who eat real ingredients who really have to worry about counting calories or carbs or fats.

Every good carpenter has a bag full of tools. A good healthcare provider should certainly be in yours. Remember, however, that your doctor does not replace your need to become educated or to be proactive in your health. Doctors can be vital in emergencies, but often are not equipped to help you rebuild your health.

Suppose your house catches on fire today.

Who are you going to call?

That's right, the fire department. They're going to

come, and they're going to bring big water hoses and lots of water, and axes. They're going to chop into the walls, and squirt water, and they're going to perform many heroics that are going to perhaps save your house. Maybe your kitchen and the garage burn down, but the bedroom and the back of the house were all saved. We're certainly glad that the firefighters were there; they are America's finest.

However, the next day, when your house is already halfway burned down, are you going to call the fire department to come back with more fire hoses and more water and more axes?

Well, of course not! You're going to call a carpenter with hammers and nails and two-by-fours. We can't use the same tools to rebuild the house that we used to put out the fire. Likewise, in your health, emergency medicine is fabulous and second-to-none in this country. But if we rely on that same type of care to rebuild our health we will find ourselves in a world of hurt.

WE HAVE TO BECOME PROACTIVE

There are two ways we can live our lives: We can be pro-active, or we can be re-active. Reactive people tend to wait until something happens to them, and then they react to that something based upon the ideas or values that they learned previously in their lives. However, proactive people can anticipate and see things moving a certain direction, and actually prevent it. True healthcare is a proactive endeavor. Disease management, as discussed earlier, is reactive.

Imagine your child is chasing a ball, running towards the street. You see the child running, and you see a car coming down the street. A proactive person would jump up, run out there, grab the child, holler at the child, maybe even scare the child into stopping and not running out into the road, because you don't want to see your child get run over. A reactive model would be to wait until the child gets run over, and then call 911. I'm reminded of this poem about prevention written in 1895.

A Fence or an Ambulance
by Joseph Malins (1895)

'Twas a dangerous cliff, as they freely confessed,
though to walk near its crest was so pleasant;
but over its terrible edge there had slipped
a duke and full many a peasant.

So the people said something would have to be done,
but their projects did not at all tally;
some said, "Put a fence 'round the edge of the cliff,"
some, "An ambulance down in the valley."

But the cry for the ambulance carried the day,
for it spread through the neighboring city;

Ninety-Nine Percent of Your Health Happens
Outside Your Doctor's Office

a fence may be useful or not, it is true,
but each heart became full of pity
for those who slipped over the dangerous cliff;

And the dwellers in highway and alley
gave pounds and gave pence, not to put up a fence,
but an ambulance down in the valley.

"For the cliff is all right, if you're careful," they said,
"and if folks even slip and are dropping,
it isn't the slipping that hurts them so much
as the shock down below when they're stopping."

So day after day, as these mishaps occurred,
quick forth would those rescuers sally
to pick up the victims who fell off the cliff,
with their ambulance down in the valley.

Then an old sage remarked: "It's a marvel to me
that people give far more attention
to repairing results than to stopping the cause,
when they'd much better aim at prevention.

"Let us stop at its source all this mischief," cried he,
"come, neighbors and friends, let us rally;
if the cliff we will fence, we might almost dispense
with the ambulance down in the valley."

This chapter teaches you how to be proactive:

- Physically
- Chemically
- Emotionally

Do you remember Jack LaLanne?

He spent thirty-four years on television showing us all how to live a healthy lifestyle. Jack LaLanne was a specimen of health in his younger years.

Even in his nineties Jack was fulfilling his purpose and affecting many people's lives. Because Jack was proactive with his health, he was able to influence the lifestyles of millions of people. We should all strive to be a little bit more like Jack.

He died at the age of ninety-six, but Jack didn't spend ten years dying. He was alive and exercising one day, and died the next. Because Jack took care of his health, he was able to be actively involved with his wife, kids, grandkids, and great-grandkids right up until the end. Jack didn't experience the traditional end-of-life care of nursing homes, bedpans, multiple medications, and diaper changes. He was here one day and gone the next. That's what I want for me.

How about you?

> *I'm amazed at how much better my mood is when I exercise.*
> *I haven't really done any in the last four decades. Now I am*
> *following your program and I feel great most all of the time.*
> *Thanks for challenging me.*
>
> ~ *Vanessa D.*

Become Physically Proactive

When we talk about physical health, most people think in terms of exercise. Absolutely, exercise is important, and in our programs there are very specific ways that we teach and train exercise. However, just physically moving your body more than you are now is going to be beneficial to most people.

In our society, more people sit at desk jobs, work on paperwork, and work on computers than ever before. As a nation, we're not nearly as active as we once were. If you look at an old black-and-white photo of your family — or just get on Google and find somebody else's — you're going to see a lot of skinny people.

Much of the population had farms and ranches, and we labored. We would wake up when the sun came up, and we would labor until the sun went down, and then we would go back inside with our families. In today's world, we spend the vast majority of our time inside, not moving. Motion is life. If we don't have motion, we start to lose life.

Imagine walking through a desert, coming upon a fork in the road, and off to one side, if you go in that direction, you see a beautiful oasis and a flowing river. Off to the other side, you see a stagnant pond.

Which direction would you take?

Most of us would go toward that flowing river, because the movement of the water filters it as the water goes over the rocks. Motion is an important factor in how water purifies itself, whereas a stagnant pond would be full of many things that would be detrimental to us. We have to learn to move more.

Many people ask, "Well, how should I exercise?"

I can't give you a specific answer in this book, because what works for one person may not work for another. There are some very specific ways to exercise that we teach to our practice members depending on their individual lab work, history, condition, etc. My job in this book is to help you understand why it's important to move your body physically.

Find ways to put physical activity into your daily lifestyle:

- Lifting weights
- Dancing
- Swimming
- Taking a water aerobics class
- Playing tennis

Whatever it is that you find enjoyable, we need to find a way to move your body more. Motion is life. Start moving more today and you will start living more today.

CAUTION: Don't overdo this one. With our practice members we usually don't start vigorous exercise for at least three months because we must first lay the foundation of healthy brain, hormone, and digestive function. Many people fail at their exercise program because they try to do it without first establishing the proper foundation.

Become Chemically Proactive

When it comes to chemical health, most people think of it in terms of: *What I'm putting into my body.*

Remember that you are what you absorb, whether you're absorbing it through your intestines or absorbing it through your skin. In chemical health, we have to look at our nutrition, and we have to evaluate what we're putting into our bodies, but we're also going to have to take time and look at what are we putting on our skin.

Consider the products you use regularly, products like:

- Shampoos, conditioners
- Shaving creams
- Lotions
- Household cleansers

- Medications
- Perfumes, colognes
- Packaged foods
- Fruits and vegetables

Are they full of chemicals and pesticides?

Many people are polluting their internal environment each and every day of their lives with prescription or over-the-counter medications.

A study done by the Environmental Working Group in 2005 looked at infant umbilical cord blood and found 287 chemicals in these infants. That means that even before a child is born into this world they already have 287 industrial chemicals flowing through their tiny bodies! Of the 287 chemicals detected in umbilical cord blood, we know that 180 of them cause cancer in humans or animals, 217 are toxic to the brain and nervous system, and 208 cause birth defects or abnormal development in animal tests. We live in a society that's full of chemical burdens, and if we want true health it's time we recognize it.

In my talks, I often ask people, "What's the number-one cause of liver toxicity?"

More often than not, I hear alcoholism; however, the number one cause of liver toxicity in the United States is the chemical burden placed on us by the medications that we're taking to make us "healthy." Tylenol (Acetaminophen) accounts for more than

56,000 emergency room visits, 2,600 hospitalizations, and an estimated **458 deaths** due to acute liver failure each year.

If we are going to maximize our health potential we need to become more aware of what we're putting into our bodies in the form of:

- Food
- Drink
- Medications
- Toothpaste
- Tampons and sanitary napkins
- Clothing

It's not only about nutrition. We also have to become aware of our environment and where we live. We must begin to look at detoxifying our bodies and we need to be proactive with our chemical burden.

> *My body hasn't felt this great in years.*
> ~ *Erica J.*

Become Emotionally Proactive

Emotional stress is rampant in our society. As a culture, we tend to be very, very busy. There are many cultures in which people take time to slow down and relax during the day, but that's not the American way.

We have phrases to describe this:

"I have too many irons in the fire."

"I'm burning my candle at both ends."

Most of us have forgotten how to slow down and invest in our emotional health. We're too busy taking the kids to soccer practice, band practice, this recital and that game, and all the while, we're expected to show up at work every day and do a good job, and participate fully. These emotional stresses can cause significant changes to your body's hormones.

The only time I hear stress being discussed in the medical community is after somebody's had a heart attack. Doctors do a lot of tests but can't find out why the person had a heart attack. The best modern medicine has to offer can't find anything wrong.

The patient is just told, "Well, maybe it's stress. You should get a hobby."

But stress is what caused the heart attack.

According to Alan Gertler, MD, associate professor of medicine in UAB's Division of Cardiovascular Diseases, "The first manifestation of a heart problem oftentimes is sudden death."[2]

Think about that: The first sign of the disease (caused by stress) is death.

2   https://www.uab.edu/news/youcanuse/item/2051-masked-heart-problems-in-men-could-lead-to-sudden-death

A third of our population is taking some type of medication for their digestive problems accounting for over $10 billion dollars a year in revenue for the drug companies. Millions of people are taking medications for high blood pressure, all of which are directly associated with emotional stress and trauma. If we want to be proactive in our health, we can't leave out this vital component. We must become proactive with our emotional health.

I want you to stop what you are doing right now and begin to think of how you are going to become proactive physically, chemically, and emotionally. Let's start with baby steps.

Chapter Three Action Items

1. Ask yourself who has been making your health decisions. Was it you, your spouse, another family member, or your doctor? Have you outsourced your decision-making?

2. Navigate to www.familyfocuswellnesscenter.com/live Print and fill in Your Wellness Score.

3. Share your answers with someone else. Remember we are much more accountable and therefore much more successful when we involve someone else and ask for their support. If you need help filling out the worksheet, or if you want us to review your answers, or if you have any questions, email me at dradams@ familyfocuswellnesscenter.com.

CHAPTER FOUR

Bringing Your Team Together

> *I feel great, but more importantly, I just feel at peace again. My anxiety is totally gone and so are those horrible medications. Thank you.*
>
> *~ Beatrice R.*

DESIGNING YOUR HEALTHCARE TEAM

Most people find their healthcare provider either as a referral from another doctor, or from a random internet search. Very little thought goes into finding a doctor. The doctor you choose is going to make a critical difference in the type of results you achieve and the quality of life that you have. This section is about establishing your own healthcare team, how to do that, and why it's important to your outcome.

Why You Need a Team

If you look at any professional sports team, there are many people who have many different talents, but it's the combination of those talents that creates a winning team. Some may be taller, some may be shorter, some may be faster, some may be stronger, but it's the dynamics of all of these different body types and skill sets put together that can create that winning outcome. No individual is able to be all things and do all things.

The same is true in our healthcare. Most people have a primary care provider, and then that primary care doctor refers you to specialists. Very few people ever take the time to interview who that primary care doctor is going to be. Professional teams spend thousands—if not tens of thousands—of dollars on recruiting, to make sure that they get the right personnel to fit the right position. Yet I find most people never really take the time to interview their doctor prior to putting them on their team.

If your health is your most important asset, which I believe it should be, then I think it's imperative that you take time to put your team together. Building the proper team will give you the best chance to create optimum health. I would never go to a doctor's appointment without first interviewing that doctor to find out if we are a good fit. However, this happens every single day, and if you ask to interview a doctor, and they're not willing to give you their time, then to me, that would tell me all I need to know. I would be looking elsewhere. Not only is it okay, but it should be expected that we interview our doctors before allowing them into our lives and into our bodies.

How to Pick Your Team

When putting your healthcare team together, I think you need to work with people you can connect with.

Look for practitioners you:

- Enjoy
- Can relate to
- Can talk with

I certainly don't think that your healthcare provider should be your best friend; on the other hand, I do think that you should be able to get along with them and come to agreements with them regarding your decision-making process. Far too many generations have just done whatever the doctor said, and doctor's orders were golden.

I think it's important to understand that you are the coach of your healthcare team. You need to be in control. Just because you're referred to Dr. Jones down the street, doesn't mean she's the one you have to see.

There's a great number of surgeons out there, and quite frankly, some are better than others. If I were being referred for surgery, I would want to meet the doctor prior to the surgery.

I would want to be able to talk to some of their patients who had the same surgery and ask them:

What was your outcome?

Was it a positive experience?

Would you use that surgeon again?

That last question is the most important one. Unfortunately, with healthcare and HIPAA regulations today, it's more and more difficult to get answers, but prior to undergoing any life-changing procedures, I would certainly ask friends and family and find out if anybody has experience with that particular doctor.

Today we are fortunate enough to have the internet, where we can look at the websites of the doctors and their practices. There are plenty of websites out there that grade doctors, clinics, and hospitals. If we take a little time on the front end to do our homework, we can expect better care and outcomes on the back end. One important thing to remember is that just because a doctor has one negative review doesn't necessarily mean that she or he's a bad doctor.

I recall looking for a pediatrician for our special-needs daughter. I called several pediatricians' offices and asked them for an interview. If they weren't willing to allow me to interview them, then I already knew that they were not a good choice for our family and our daughter.

The physician who did allow me to interview him gave me a half-hour of his time. I know he's very busy, and I was very appreciative of that. We had an open discussion about what our expectations would be, and he agreed to those expectations, and we began a wonderful long-term relationship.

The first one I interviewed hadn't work out so well. We fired that doctor. It is okay to kick people off your team. It *is* okay to fire your doctor.

Finding a Mentor

Our healthcare system in this country is broken. The biggest thing that's missing is mentoring. It's not your doctor's fault that (based on the national average) they may be able to give you only about seven to nine minutes per visit. You may have a great doctor. I'm not blaming them or beating them up. But the system is designed for practitioners to see more and more people, just to be able to keep the lights on.

Doctors used to spend more time with their patients:

- Giving advice
- Mentoring
- Educating

Now that's been replaced with, "What pharmacy do you use? Here's your prescription."

We need to get back to a time of the family doctor who really took the time to discuss with you other aspects of your health, including:

- Diet
- Fitness level
- Lifestyle choices

If you really want to have optimum function, you need to find a doctor who's willing to mentor you.

All successful people—in life and business—use mentors. Mentors are people who are in your sphere of influence who have more knowledge in a particular subject than you do and are excited to share that knowledge and education with you. All successful athletes and all successful businessmen have mentors or coaches who help them excel in their particular sport or field of study. If you want to excel in your health, you need to find a good mentor.

We should all look for that coach or that mentor in our doctor. The word "doctor" is the agentive noun of the Latin verb *docere* (do-ke-re), which means "to teach." Very few doctors are teaching in today's healthcare environment. Doctors don't have time to teach and educate the way that they could two or three decades ago.

In searching for a doctor to put on your team, you want to find somebody who:

- Educates
- Explains
- Helps you discover how to return to optimum function

Don't settle for someone who just wants to hand out some pills to reduce symptoms and see you again in six months.

I remember when my son was playing high school baseball. There were 18 sixteen- and seventeen-year-old boys on his team.

If the coach didn't show up to practice, what do you think those boys would be doing?

Well, of course, they would be chasing girls.

When the coach arrived, he'd take control and help the boys understand that they needed to practice throwing, batting, fielding, and running. He was an effective mentor. Coaches who mentor effectively are most often the ones who lead their teams to win the championship.

When it comes to your health, there's nothing more important than winning; therefore, you want to make sure that you have a good coach or mentor. When you are tired of chasing symptoms and you are ready to optimize your health, contact me at:

dradams@familyfocuswellnesscenter.com

I would love to be a part of your team.

> *My cholesterol dropped ninety points when I followed the program you put me on. I was able to get off three blood pressure drugs and two cholesterol-lowering drugs. It is so frustrating that I wasted the last sixteen years feeling terrible because my doctor wouldn't take the time to actually show me how to take my life back. Thank you giving me the tools and education to take my life back.*
>
> ~ *Geraldine F.*

TAKING RESPONSIBILITY

I'm not sure when it happened, but at some point, the vast majority of Americans quit taking responsibility for their own health. We've been trained and educated to believe that we just live our lives until something goes wrong, then we go to our doctor and expect them to fix it.

Our bodies are self-healing and self-regulating creations. You're going to have to recognize that and take responsibility for your own body if you want to function and live seven, eight, nine, or even ten decades in optimum health.

What Is Your Role?

What role should you play on your healthcare team?

You are the coach. You're the one who calls all the shots.

Understand and educate yourself on any recommendations from your doctor, such as:

- Potential treatments
- Procedures
- Medications
- Diagnostic testing
- Surgery

I'm not saying that you need to be as knowledgeable as your doctor and you certainly don't need to go to twelve years of medical school, but you should be well informed about the recommended procedures. Weigh the risks and the benefits, and if you decide that the benefits outweigh the risks, then move forward with that particular treatment or approach. However, if you decide that the risks outweigh the benefits, then you should recognize that just because the doctor recommended it doesn't mean that it has to happen.

Our daughter Ashley was prescribed a surgery that entailed removing a large part of her skull. We weighed the risks and the benefits, and as a family we decided that it probably wasn't worth the risks. We elected a different form of treatment.

What we chose to do instead of the surgery cleared up the problem within a couple of weeks, and we didn't have to remove a large part of her skull. However, if we had just taken the recommendations of the first person we saw, then we would have opted for the surgery. You're the first advocate for yourself as well as your children, even before the doctor. Go with your own best judgment, based on the recommendations that you're given.

When my first child was born, we were fairly young parents and fairly clueless as to what was going on. Our son had a tear in his neck caused by the birthing process. This caused his head to lean and turn to one side, a condition called *torticollis*. It was recommended to us that we leave it this way until age twelve, at which time a surgery would be done to sever the muscles of the neck and straighten it out. Even as young parents who knew very little, we knew that this just didn't sound right.

We got a second opinion, and as a result, with three months of care from a pediatric chiropractor, he was completely balanced and corrected and no longer required surgery. Now he is a college baseball player chasing his dreams. If we had followed the advice of the first physician, he wouldn't have been able to pursue his passion.

> *Thank you for all you have done to improve my life.*
> *~ Rhonda W.*

Knowing the Score

When talking to patients, one of the things that really

bothers me is that very few people know the score. Most of my practice members have some general idea of treatments they've done, or surgeries they've had, but they're really relatively uninformed as to any other specifics. A good example would be that patients will go in for their routine visit; they'll have blood labs done and they'll hear nothing back.

Two or three weeks later they finally call the clinic and they ask, "How did my labs turn out?"

After you are placed on hold for twenty minutes, someone will get back on the phone only to say, "Oh, your labs all looked good," and that's the end of the conversation.

If you're going to take the time and effort to get blood labs done, then you certainly should expect your doctor to take the time to explain those results to you. You should get a copy of the results with an explanation of each item. It's imperative that you get copies of reports for any procedure, any test, anything that's ever done on or to you. Add them to a file of your health records that you maintain.

If your doctor isn't giving these to you and explaining them in detail and answering all your questions, then you probably don't have the right doctor. I usually spend at least thirty minutes with each of my practice members to explain to them exactly what their lab results reveal.

I recall speaking to a gentleman, a healthcare provider, who sat in my office as a patient. He shared with me that he worked for a doctor in a clinic.

The first two weeks he was there, the doctor handed him a stack of labs and said, "Here, call all of these people, and tell them their labs are normal."

He said the one on the top of his giant stack had two or three "H"s for "high"s and two or three "L"s for "low"s.

He asked the doctor, "Well, what about this?"

The doctor said, "Just call them and tell them they're normal."

The man proceeded to make about fifty calls to patients and told everybody that their labs were normal, when in actuality there were quite a few things that were wrong.

You need to get a copy of your own labs, your own X-rays, MRIs, surgery notes, and so on. If there is something you do not understand, talk to your primary care physician, or surgeon, or whoever performed or asked for that particular test, and ask them to take the time to explain it. If they're not willing to take the time to explain the results of the tests and what they mean, then in my opinion, those practitioners should not be on your team.

When patients bring bloodwork into my office, if they do happen to have a copy, it's usually one, maybe two pages, maximum. The blood results that we go over with our patients are usually twenty to twenty-four pages, because we take the time to explain what all of those individual values mean. I think it's important to know your score.

Winning the Game

Now that we've built a good team and we have a great coach, it's time to win the game.

When it comes to your health or your quality of life, what is winning?

That's not for me to define. That's for you to define.

However, I think most people have a few goals in common:

- To grow old gracefully
- To have truly golden Golden Years
- Not just going from one doctor's visit to another
- To be independent of drugs and medications
- To be fully present with our families and friends

Most people generally don't enjoy going to the doctor. My definition of winning the game would be staying out of the doctor's offices. All too often, when people get into their seventies and eighties, the vast majority of their time outside of the house is spent in a doctor's office. My version of winning the game is never having to see a doctor because I have a problem, only visiting one to prevent problems.

I recently heard a doctor from the Cleveland Clinic say he and most of his colleagues have never seen a healthy patient. We call it healthcare, but it is really disease management. I think it's really sad that most doctors don't see healthy patients.

If you properly assemble a team—designing your healthcare team—and begin being proactive with your health, you should only be seeing your doctors to help you stay healthy, not get healthy. It should be the rare exception that you see them in cases of crisis, sickness, illness, or disease. Take a few moments to define what winning the game looks like for you.

The World Health Organization defines health as, "...a state of complete physical, mental, and social well-being, not merely the absence of disease or infirmity."[3]

Being just not-sick is not good enough. Optimum health means optimum body function.

The most important takeaway, hopefully, from this chapter is that you understand that if you begin to take more responsibility for your choices, you will end up with a higher quality of life. When you take responsibility for your decisions and healthcare, you will end up with a higher quality of life and stronger relationships.

---

[3] http://www.who.int/about/definition/en/print.html

Ultimately, I think that's what it's all about: Our quality of life, and our relationships. I've never seen a hearse with a U-Haul. It's not about the amount of things that we collect, but it's how we interact with people and the impact that we leave with our family, our community, and in our world that matters. It all starts with taking responsibility for your own body and health.

> *Thank you for empowering me to take control of my own health. You and your team are amazing!*
>
> *~ Lester S.*

THE BEST WAY TO LEARN IS TO TEACH

The best way to learn something is to teach it. I know in college, human anatomy was a very difficult course for many people, so I picked up a tutoring job to teach people anatomy. I actually became quite good at it, because I was learning it as I was teaching it. If you've ever taught somebody something — a class, or a child — you know that you become an expert at it while teaching it.

Sharing Your Story

Everybody has a story. Everybody has a journey. Everybody has experiences. We all have something to learn from one another. Often I meet people who feel they aren't very exciting or don't have a lot to offer.

But if they open up and connect on an emotional level, I find that I can learn a tremendous amount from them.

Becoming a mentor is really nothing more than being able to open up and share your personal experiences and stories in a very real, raw, and relevant way that can have an impact on others.

We've all done things; we all know things. We've all experienced things that others haven't. As we learn to share our experiences, and share with others, not only can we have an impact on them, but we're also helping ourselves.

Impacting Others

I recommend that my practice members share their experiences.

I encourage them to share how they have become:

- More educated
- More self-reliant
- Better able to make decisions concerning their health

Many of the things I've found that work for me and my family came from other people who were willing to share. As we become more educated and we share with others, it solidifies our experience and it helps to make a positive influence on those we care about and those around us.

The world of healthcare seems to be a very independent world:

- One doctor
- One patient
- One experience

However, if we look at other experiences in life, such as education, we tend to do this in a classroom setting. We don't have one teacher and one student, but it's the dynamics of the group. Everybody has something to offer that leads to some of the greatest educational experiences or learning opportunities.

In my professional practice as a physician, during the first fifteen years of practice, everything I did was one-on-one; I met with one patient at a time. Then, in 2014, I began to put groups of patients with similar experiences or similar conditions together. I began to put people together in groups, with their permission, and we began to do education in a group setting.

What I discovered was the dynamics of the group were so much more powerful than mine as an individual. Not only did my patients get more out of their appointments, but also we were able to spend more time — because we were in a group setting — so we could get deeper into lifestyle modifications.

I've learned a tremendous amount from my patients, and my patients have been able to share with one another, so that we all have impacted one another.

> *Dr. Adams, you're making a huge change in your community. I'm really impressed with that.*
>
> ~ *Dr. Charles Webb*
> *International Speaker, Author of Metamorphosis*

Leaving a Legacy

One of your greatest possible achievements is knowing that you are a blessing to someone else. Ultimately, if you are only in this life for yourself and what you can get for yourself, something is very much missing. Even though you may not be a firefighter, paramedic, healthcare provider, or a teacher, you can still have a significant impact on someone else's life or someone else's experience.

In high school they brought in guest speakers to tell us not to do drugs. Every one of those speakers had been on drugs, lived on the streets, been homeless, and really had a horrible experience. Those speakers made good use of a horrible situation; if they had never had that experience, they wouldn't be very effective at helping kids avoid those pitfalls.

As human beings, we are all connected, and should be connecting with others, and sharing the knowledge that we have. As you share your life with others you are leaving a legacy.

Chapter Four Action Items

1. Do you have a healthcare team or some disease-management doctors? Decide today that you are going to be the coach of a winning team. Assemble your players (healthcare providers), and make certain that you are setting yourself up to win the game.

2. Navigate to www.familyfocuswellnesscenter.com/live Print and fill in the "Are you winning the game?" worksheet.

3. Print several of these to share with your friends and family and ask if they are winning the game. Of course if you want us to review your answers, have any questions, or need help filling it out, email me at dradams@ familyfocuswellnesscenter.com.

CHAPTER FIVE

Designing Your Future

DESIGNING YOUR HEALTH

Most people spend a significant amount of time, energy, and investment on planning out their lives:

- They'll spend four years in college to find out what type of career they'd like to have.
- They will spend countless hours finding the right home.
- They spend time picking and choosing their spouses
- They plan their families.
- They plan retirements.

But very few people spend any time planning their health, or designing their health.

Health is our most important asset. If it's true that, as we often hear, without health we have nothing, why is this one aspect of our lives that we spend little to no time planning for and designing?

This chapter is about how to design your future.

Where Do You Want to Be?

If you don't do anything differently than you're currently doing, where do you see yourself in the next three to five years?

I ask this question of all the practice members who come into our office and often get responses like:

- On a walker
- In a wheelchair
- In a nursing home
- Dead

As time moves by, it's really true that most people do not get healthier. We're only aging and getting older, and if you are not designing your future, then the only way you will go is downhill.

However, with proper lifestyle design—by designing your health—you can actually be younger three to five years from now than you are today. You may not be chronologically younger, but as far as your health is concerned, you can definitely feel amazing if you implement the proper design.

Another set of questions I like to ask is:

If you could see yourself one year from now, what would you want your life to look like?

- More energy?
- Better digestion?
- Decreased pain?
- Decreased inflammation?
- Balanced hormones?
- Clearer thinking?
- Reversal of your disease process?

Would you like to get off of some of those prescription drugs that you've been on for years?

Would you like to improve your libido?

Improve your relationships and your quality of life?

All of these things are possible one year from now, if you make changes, if you design your future and implement that plan.

If ten birds are sitting on a fence and one decides to fly south for the winter, how many birds are left on the fence?

The answer is ten. Just because one *decided* to fly south doesn't mean the bird actually did.

Just deciding to change your lifestyle won't be enough; you *must* take action in order to get results. I've often heard that if we fail to plan, we plan to fail.

Are you planning to fail, or are you planning to truly transform your future?

> *Since being on your program I have not only lost forty-eight pounds but have been able to keep it off for over three years now. Thank you for explaining how it was truly a hormone problem, not a weight problem. And thank you for showing me how to balance my hormones. I am a better mother and wife now.*
> ~ Rebecca M.

Breaking Free of a Broken System

As discussed earlier in this book, most of us are currently in a broken healthcare system. It isn't providing healthcare at all; it's just providing sick care management.

If you want to continue to manage your sickness and illness, then that's a great system and you should keep doing what you're doing. But if you want different results, you have to do something different. The something different I'm challenging you to do is to break free of that broken system.

You need to gain independence over your health. Ninety-nine percent of healthcare should be self-care. I'm in no way saying that you should never have a primary care doctor, or that you shouldn't use the healthcare system, because it's very good at emergency care. In emergency situations, I'm so thankful it's there.

However, if you are going to design your future, then you need to recognize that you have the ability to break free of that sick care management, and embrace self-care and take responsibility for your own health.

Making Your Golden Years Golden

How would you like to spend seven, eight, nine, even ten decades of optimal health?

What's the key word?

Optimal.

How would you like to prevent the inevitable as you grow older, of ending up fat, sick, and generally depressed?

The sad truth is, when we're younger, we have a vision of our golden years being golden; however, the vast majority of people that I speak to in their sixties and beyond have come to realize that there's nothing golden about it.

Americans are working longer and longer, into their older years. Elders are putting off retirement. By the time they finally do achieve retirement, they're spending more time going to doctor's visits, seeing one specialist after another, only to be placed on one prescription after another and not really finding the gold in the golden years.

You don't want to take the luxury of waiting until you

are sick to decide that now you are going to take your health seriously. You need to make that decision before you ever become ill. You can start today making those decisions. And if you already are into your golden years, it's not too late for you, either. It's time for you to take your health seriously, make the changes that you know that you need to make, so that you can enjoy your golden years. I recall working with an eighty-eight-year-old client who, after completing our program, said she felt like she was in her forties again.

I've heard it said, "I'm not afraid of dying; I'm afraid of living too long."

Most Americans are spending their last ten to fifteen years in a nursing home, wondering why the kids and grandkids don't come visit them. Let's make sure you're not one of those people.

> *At eighty-eight and eighty-five, we really thought that this was the way we were going to be the rest of our lives. Thank you for showing us that we weren't too old to get better. We feel like we are in our sixties again.*
> *~ Dan and Gina T.*

DESIGNING YOUR RELATIONSHIPS

The diagnosis we receive is probably about the least important part of the process.

What really matters is: How is that health problem going to affect your quality of life and your relationships?

We spend way too much time being concerned with, "What is the diagnosis?" and always coming up with newer, fancier equipment that costs tens of thousands of dollars for procedures to tell us what we have.

The more important question we need to answer is how does what we have interfere with what we experience with our families, in our work, in our hobbies, and in our life?

Let's talk about designing our relationships.

Personal Connections

I have beautiful people in my life, and so do you. People rely on me. I know people in my world who are very important to me, and I'm very important to them. You do as well. We all do.

Relationships are what makes the world a special place. I have spent a lot of time talking about health and restoring optimum function to your health, but it's never been about a selfish endeavor.

It's been about allowing you to be the best:

- Mother
- Father
- Brother
- Sister

- Spouse
- Employee
- Employer
- Aunt
- Uncle
- Friend
- Co-worker

If you feel good all the time, you're much more fun to be around, and you can provide much more to all of those personal connections.

I recall when my daughter had her transplant procedures, she and my wife lived in a hospital 704 miles away for nearly two years. We spent a lot of conversations on the phone talking about the care, the decisions, the medications, the therapy, all of the things that were being done to save her life, but the hardest part of the entire process was the disconnections caused by the distance.

I sat next to my daughter in the hospital bed during one of our visits and said, "We've got to get her home."

We laid out a plan to get her home, because what was missing in that hospital room was her father, her brother, her sister, and her grandparents. All the technical procedures and heroics that were done to save her life were absolutely necessary, but she certainly wasn't going to thrive in that environment.

Once she was back in her home, she began to heal

and improve significantly more because not only did she have her mother, but she also had her father, her brother, her sister, her grandparents, relatives, and friends. Those personal connections are the most important part of the healing process.

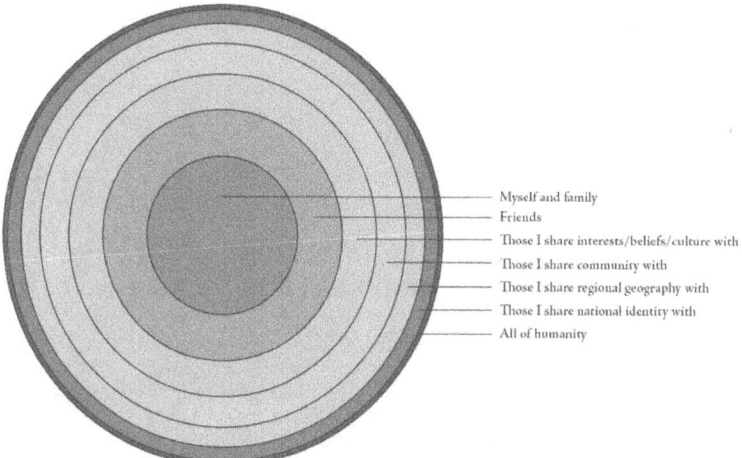

Myself and family
Friends
Those I share interests/beliefs/culture with
Those I share community with
Those I share regional geography with
Those I share national identity with
All of humanity

If you don't have yourself in order at the center of this diagram, then there's no way that you can really be the best mother, father, brother, or sister for your family. There's no way that you can fully impact your friends. If you want to make a difference in this world, it starts with you getting serious with yourself and making certain you take care of you so you can be there for them.

> *I am spending more time with my family and my kids. Now that I feel better I think I am being a better wife and mother. Thanks for helping me not suffer. I'm feeling so much more alive. I sleep like a baby and wake up feeling refreshed. And I'm not taking any more medications. I can't even remember the last time I took a Tylenol.*
>
> *~ Betty M*

Community Involvement

Have you ever been on an airplane, and paid attention to the flight attendant as they were describing the oxygen mask falling from the ceiling in the case of an emergency?

The line they always use is, "If you are traveling with a child or someone who requires assistance, secure your mask first, and then assist the other person."

To a parent, this seems counterintuitive because we are biologically designed to protect our children, but this illustrates that if we're not taking care of ourselves first, then it's less likely that we'll be able to save them.

Now let's take that out to the next ring. If I don't have my house in order, am I really going to be interacting with my extended family as well?

Or am I just going to be the one that, when we get together, talks about all my health problems and all the challenges I have?

How can I help my brother or my sister, if I don't have my own house in order?

Finally, once we have those rings in order, we can start to talk about becoming involved in the community.

If you're so sick and tired that you can't get out of your house, how are you going to be able to give to those people in your community who are needy?

How are you going to be able to keep up with volunteering?

If you feel lousy, you certainly can't. If you want to make a difference in your community, you have to take care of yourself first.

Impacting the World

Everybody has a purpose in life. As a public speaker, I address crowds on a regular basis.

Often I ask the crowd, "How many of you believe that we all have a purpose in life?"

Every hand is raised.

My follow-up question is, "How many of you are living your purpose?"

Very few people raise their hands.

Where's the disconnect?

If we all know that we have a purpose, and very few of

us are actually living that purpose, that's not okay! If you're not living your purpose, then you're not making as much of an impact on the world as you should be.

Earlier in the book I mention Jack Lalanne. He is no longer with us; he died at the age of ninety-six. However, Jack had a purpose, and his purpose was to affect people's lives by teaching them about nutrition, health, and wellness.

In his younger years, Jack was a bodybuilder and had television shows where he taught people how to exercise. In his later years, as the "Juice Man," he produced and promoted a juicer. Jack had an effect on millions of people across this planet. Because he took care of his health, he was able to have an impact on the health of millions of other people. Even though he's been gone for a number of years now, he's still fulfilling his purpose and still impacting the world through the legacy that he left. Jack took care of his health first, so that he could make that impact on the rest of us.

How are you going to impact the world?

Jack didn't spend ten years dying. He didn't live his years in a nursing home; he just died one day. That's what I hope for myself. I think most people hope for the same, rather than spending that last ten years with multiple surgeries, interventions, expenses, nursing homes, assisted living, and those kind of things.

GET OUT OF THE BOOK AND INTO YOUR LIFE

Almost everyone I've ever consulted with in my office has told me that they've read a health book or a diet book in the past, yet here they are in my office, on a number of different medications with a number of different diagnoses and a number of different problems.

Why is that?

Because *reading a book will not make you healthy!*

Many of the things that you've read throughout this book are probably things that you've already heard before. There's really not a whole lot of new concepts that we've discussed. What's going to make it different for you this time is if you let us help get you out of the book and into your life. In the following sections, we're really going to spend some time to help you design your:

- Future
- Relationships
- Health
- Life

As we go through the following sections, I don't want you to just read this chapter. I want you to have a pen, paper, and an internet connection. We are going to get you out of the book and start changing your life right now.

> *My headaches are gone, my meds are gone, and my problems are gone. You guys are the best.*
>
> ~ *Velma Y.*

Where Do I Start?

Congratulations, you've made it this far into the book.

We're going to start taking action right now. With anything new we do in life, the hardest part is getting started. I want you to commit to yourself that sometime within the next forty-eight hours you will schedule some time to do the action items at the ends of Chapters One through Four.

If you haven't already done them, then stop procrastinating and get to work. Go to www. familyfocuswellnesscenter.com/live and download the worksheets. If you have already done them, then congratulations! You are the type of person who takes action and they always get the best results.

If you're a current practice member, please bring the completed worksheets by the office and we'll review them together. If you're not a current member and you would like to learn more, feel free to email your results to me at DrAdams@FamilyFocusWellnessCenter. com, and I will be happy to set up a complimentary consultation to review them with you.

What Do I Do?

Now that you've completed the worksheets, where do you go from here?

Start by making a list. Most people are used to the idea of going to a doctor and telling them what's wrong, and telling them what they don't want.

For instance:

"I don't want this headache."

"I don't want these digestive problems."

"I don't want this high blood pressure and high cholesterol."

But we spend very little time talking about what we *do* want.

So make a list of the things that you do want.

Instead of writing, "I don't want pain," what's the opposite of that?

Perhaps you could write:

"I do want freedom of mobility."

"I do want to be able to roll around on the floor with my grandkids."

"I do want to be able to sit through a movie without having to get up and walk around because I'm hurting."

"I do want to be able to enjoy my relationships more."

Instead of writing, "I don't want to have high cholesterol," you could write, "I do want to have healthy, functioning cholesterol levels."

Instead of writing, "I don't want high blood pressure," write, "I do want to have optimum blood pressure."

Instead of writing, "I don't want diabetes," write, "I do want healthy blood sugar levels and a healthy heart."

I want you to begin by making a list, not of the things that you don't want, but of the things that you would do if you could have your optimum health.

To help get you thinking, some of the most common things that we see in our office are:

"I want improved digestion, more energy, increased libido, more stamina."

"I want more self confidence."

"I want to be able to look in the mirror and like who I see."

"I want to finally get rid of these prescriptions."

Go get started making your list!

Now that you have your list, we need to turn that list into a plan. I would highly recommend finding a mentor to help hold you accountable to make sure you implement your plan. If you don't have a mentor, or if you would like more information, please contact me.

Living in the Journey

Health is a journey, not a destination. If we've had a health problem for a few weeks, months, years or decades, it's unrealistic to expect it to go away overnight. Many people quit their diets because they don't see immediate results. Most people see their health as a series of events: the time that they broke their ankle or had their gall bladder removed or were diagnosed with cancer.

However, health is not a series of events, but rather, a journey. By taking the time to fill out the worksheets found at www.familyfocuswellnesscenter.com/live and reflecting on your answers, you will be well on your way to turning your life around. But it is important that you recognize that it will take some time to see results.

As Americans, we have a microwave mentality that says, "I want it, and I want it now!" which is why we have such a drug-dependent culture that treats our symptoms and ignores the underlying problem.

Please recognize that in order to have optimum health and function, so that we can have that incredible quality of life and very deep, connected relationships, you need to invest time and effort into this process.

You were given an amazing body that is capable of healing itself in very big ways within a relatively short period of time. If you make small changes, you'll get small outcomes, but if you're ready to make a big change you can expect a big outcome.

Once you begin the correct program of lifestyle changes you can expect to see results very early on. I'm always astounded at how quickly people are able to reverse their diabetes or restore their hormones to balance. I'm amazed at how quickly people are able to normalize their blood pressure, get off of their cholesterol medications, improve their energy levels, lose significant amounts of weight, improve their stamina, self-worth, and self image.

I encourage you not to use this book as another short-term quick fix, but to really take the concepts learned and make them part of your lifestyle. If you want long-term results, you need to make long-term changes. I'm asking you to not just take the concepts in this book and follow them temporarily, because you will get temporary results at best. I'm asking you to do this not only for yourself, so that your golden years can be golden, but so that you can have an impact on generations to come.

Have you heard of the starfish story?

All the starfish have washed up on the beach, and some kid is gathering them up and throwing them back in.

Somebody comes along and looks at the kid and says, "There are too many starfish! You're not going to make a difference."

The kid picks up a starfish, tosses it into the ocean, and says, "It made a difference for that one."

I want you to start with yourself. Make a difference for you so that you can make a difference for all those people who love you.

Dr. Adams, I appreciate how you explain every topic you are trying to help me understand. This shows how much you care that we get it. Many times, a doctor just recites a short scripted reply and hands over a prescription. Your approach is straightforward as well as informational. I am looking forward to great results with the excellent care of your staff and yourself. Thank you.

~ Dee M.

Chapter Five Action Items

1. Schedule time right now to make your list. List what you really want to gain, not just what do you want to get rid of.

2. Navigate to www.familyfocuswellnesscenter.com/live Print and fill out "What Do I Want to Gain." Read "As Your Doctor," "10 Objections," and "Can You Afford to Be Healthy?"

3. Read the report, "Stress, Hormones, and Belly Fat," and share it with your friends.

4. If you haven't attended one of my live events and would like to, call 903-236-6222 and find out when and where our next Live event will be held.

5. If you would like us to do an event for your company, church group, civic group, or other gathering, please contact us to make arrangements.

6. Share what you have learned in this book with your friends and family.

Conclusion

I've spent the better part of two decades working with people, mentoring people, talking with people about their health and their healthcare, their decisions, and where they would like to be.

One thing I've consistently discovered is that almost no one was taught to be proactive with their health. We're completely reactive. We wait until we have a problem. We wait until we have an illness, a diagnosis, a condition, before we take action, and we do this because we've been trained to do this. We've been trained to wait until we're sick, and typically very sick, where the over-the-counter stuff or Mom's home remedies don't work anymore.

We wait until we're really sick and then we expect our doctors to heal our problems. As you read though these pages, I hope you began to understand that health and healing is something that comes from within. We can no longer physically or financially afford to outsource our healthcare.

There's only one cause to all disease, and that cause is stress. The only cure is to help our bodies, support our bodies in their ability to overcome that stress. We live in a fast-paced society, a fast-paced culture. We're always going and doing, and very rarely do we slow down and take time to recognize that our bodies are doing those things for us.

My hope as you read through these pages is that you began to understand that if you want optimum health and function, and you want your golden years to be golden, then it's necessary to begin to respect that body that you were given.

I've seen patients from newborn infants to seniors well into their nineties. I have always been amazed at the human body's ability to turn itself around. I'm reminded of an eighty-eight year old patient who had never been in a gym a day in her life, wasn't really eating well and hadn't for decades. When I initially met her, I was really concerned because she just wasn't going to turn things around, but I was astonished to see that within just a few short months, she was able to regain some of her youth and vitality, and responded that she felt forty years younger!

Don't use excuses that you're too young, too old, or too tired. Don't come up with excuses to miss an opportunity. If you haven't already begun to take the actions that you've read in these pages, then certainly now is the time.

If you made it through all five chapters, then I want you to go back to the final chapter, Designing Your Future, and really commit to yourself that you're going to take the action steps required to begin to turn your body, your health, and your life around. Remember, you're not just doing this for yourself. You're doing it for those who care about you, you're doing it for your community, and you're doing it for those around you.

Earlier in the book, we discussed finding a mentor and finding someone to be accountable to. That mentor can be a good friend, it can be a spouse, it can be a family member, but often times we've found that it's best if that person is someone who's not close to you, because the people close to you won't always hold you accountable when you need them to. They'll give you a little more slack than maybe you should be willing to take.

If you haven't found a mentor, I would love to be that mentor for you. My team and I would love to be able to teach you, and show you how to gain optimal health by applying the five pillars of health to your life. In our office, we've put together a very unique and specialized program to walk people through the processes that have been discussed in this book.

I suspect there's not a whole lot in this book that you didn't already know. The problem is that you may just not be doing it. We've designed a specialized program to help people and walk people through the individual steps, to apply the five pillars of health and return to optimum function. These programs are individually designed, based upon your unique laboratory findings, hormone balance, history, and health needs or health conditions.

If you're sick and tired of being sick and tired, and you're ready to restore your life, your mind, your body, and your relationships, then contact us at:

Family Focus Wellness Center, 903-236-6222

Or feel free to ask any questions you have at:

DrAdams@FamilyFocusWellnessCenter.com

Next Steps

So what's next?

Well, that depends on you.

This can be just another book that collects dust or one that can have a lasting impact on your life and those that surround you. I would ask that if you enjoyed this book, you keep it alive by giving it to someone you care about and asking them to read and apply its concepts as well. Then, when they get to this page, hopefully they will pass it on too.

If you are ready to get your life back on track, I would love to help you.

You can contact me at:

Family Focus Wellness Center, 903-236-6222

dradams@familyfocuswellnesscenter.com

I would be honored to either help you directly or put you in touch with one of my colleagues in your area who can help you accomplish your goals.

Don't procrastinate. Call today.

About the Author

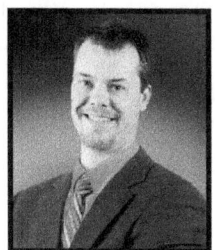

Dr. David Adams will be the first to tell you it's not the years of undergraduate, graduate, and post-graduate training that qualify him. It's not even the twenty-plus years of clinical expertise and experience that qualify him. Life qualifies him.

Through the life-and-death struggles of fathering a chronically ill child, he has learned firsthand how delicate and fragile a person's health can become. His personal experiences have shaped his life's purpose.

He says, "It is my mission to improve the quality of life and relationships in the individuals and families I am blessed to help. My goal is to assist others in getting the most out of this life. Without taking proper care of the life you are given the quality of your life can quickly slip away. Your life and your health is a gift and it's my mission to help you protect that gift."

Dr. Adams welcomes you to become one of the thousands of members of the Family Focus Wellness Center to live the healthiest, most fulfilled life possible. Together, we can correct the cause naturally rather than artificially; we can revitalize rather than numb. Dr. Adams' purpose is to help you remove the interference to the expression of your life.